Natural Therapies

for

OVERCOMING
OPIOID
DEPENDENCY

Dr. Catherine Browne
Doctor of Acupuncture and Oriental Medicine

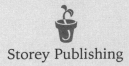
Storey Publishing

The mission of Storey Publishing is to serve our customers by
publishing practical information that encourages
personal independence in harmony with the environment.

EDITED BY Nancy Ringer and Sarah Guare
ART DIRECTION AND BOOK DESIGN BY Alethea Morrison and Erin Dawson
INDEXED BY Christine R. Lindemer, Boston Road Communications
COVER ILLUSTRATION BY © Koren Shadmi
INTERIOR ILLUSTRATIONS BY Ilona Sherratt
Author photograph courtesy of the author

This publication is intended to provide educational information for the reader on the covered subject. It is not intended to take the place of personalized medical counseling, diagnosis, and treatment from a trained health professional.

Storey books are available for special premium and promotional uses and for customized editions. For further information, please call 800-793-9396.

Storey Publishing
210 MASS MoCA Way
North Adams, MA 01247
storey.com

Printed in the United States by McNaughton & Gunn, Inc.
10 9 8 7 6 5 4 3 2 1

Library of Congress Cataloging-in-Publication Data on file

Contents

Acknowledgments

Thanks to my teachers, who have been patient, and to my patients, who have been teachers. A special thanks to my teacher Kathleen Leavy, AP, RN; she has graciously trained hundreds of acupuncturists and made the world a better place.

I hold much gratitude in my heart for Barbara Fields, RN, who took me under her wing and taught me manifestion at a higher level, allowing me to bring my dreams to fruition.

I give a special thanks to William VanNess, MD, who invited me into his opioid-free Pain and Rehab Institute. There he has been demonstrating great compassion for patients while alleviating pain without the use of narcotic drugs for decades, long before others recognized the risks of opioid addiction.

Thanks to my mother, Evelyn Padgett, who has been a fearless role model. Finally, I cannot begin to express my appreciation for my children, Emmit and Olivia, who inspire me each and every day, and for my amazingly supportive husband, Bill.

Why Consider Natural Therapies?

You, or perhaps your family and friends, may be skeptical that natural therapies could possibly be powerful enough to effectively treat opioid addiction. What sort of natural therapies could hope to compete with established medical and pharmaceutical protocols for a destructive and debilitating health condition of such epic proportions?

As it turns out, high recidivism rates for opioid users indicate that the traditional approach to addiction treatment — drug therapy (to detoxify and/or to substitute for opioids), behavioral therapy, and counseling — is not working; relapse rates are reported to be as high as 91 percent.[1] Meanwhile, an explosion of scientifically validated, peer-reviewed studies, which you can find at such venerable sources as the National Institutes of Health's PubMed database, are proving that natural therapies — treatments that use energetic healing, botanical medicines, and mindfulness to stimulate, support, and heal the body's own systems of healing — can help opioid users successfully overcome addiction, reduce withdrawal symptoms, and manage pain for the long term.

In fact, natural therapies like acupuncture, acupressure, medicinal herbs, essential oils, nutritional strategies, supplements, and meditation have been so successful in clinical applications that they are presently being integrated into the treatment programs of major hospitals across the United States. Western medical practitioners who have been frustrated with the lack of viable options for easing pain, reversing chronic disease, or combating opioid addiction have found that natural therapies can effectively address these health issues. The reasons are multifold:

- Natural modalities are effective medicine. As studies have shown, they stimulate the body's immune, endocrine, and nervous systems, among other things, and provoke a powerful healing effect.

- While pharmaceuticals are often designed to target a particular deficiency or excess, natural therapies have a broad healing impact. They can address the underlying causes of health problems. Rather than masking or correcting symptoms, they correct the root imbalance that led to the symptoms in the first place.

- Natural therapies are wonderfully restorative. They support patients not just physically but emotionally. Illness, whether acute or long-term, including addiction, is hard on the psyche, and these therapies have been proven to soothe the nerves and brighten a patient's outlook simply by virtue of their balancing and normalizing effects.

- Natural therapies have few, if any, negative side effects, and the remedies are generally less toxic and more cost-effective than prescription drugs. Acupuncture, for example, is an excellent alternative to pharmacological treatment for pain, with little risk of side effects.[2]

- Natural therapies are not addictive. In contrast, Western medications used to treat opioid addiction, such as methadone and Subutex (buprenorphine), replace opioids with another addictive substance.

- Natural therapies are effective at reducing or completely eliminating withdrawal symptoms for people who are giving up opioids.

- Following withdrawal, patients can turn to a plethora of natural therapies to fully restore their health and vitality. These treatments can also help prevent relapse; acupuncture, for example, can play an important role not only in overcoming addiction but also in preventing a return to it.[3]

A Difference in Perspective

Beyond the proven benefits of a holistic approach versus traditional treatment, there can be a very real difference between the two approaches in their perspective on addiction. In our culture, we tend to assign a certain stigma to those who become addicted to drugs. We assume some weakness in their willpower, some fault in their choices, some contamination of their character that led them to become addicts — and that will forever mark them as addicts.

Traditional 12-step programs, for example, require participants to acknowledge that they are addicts and that their addiction is a lifelong condition. The ostensible intentions are to instill a sense of humility and accountability, to build character, and to establish a foundation of self-awareness and strength. Those are all good principles, not just for addicts but for anyone, in any situation. However, the concept of addiction as a lifelong condition is outdated. Current science on neuroplasticity (which we'll discuss in chapter 1) tells us that our brain has the potential to change and heal. That is, though our brain may become wired for addiction, we can rewire it using holistic mind-body therapies to eliminate the pathways of addiction. So, contrary to much of the literature available from traditional treatment programs, addiction is actually a curable disease.

People like to say, "Once an addict, always an addict." But that perspective runs counter to Chinese medical theory and to my personal clinical experience. As a holistic practitioner, I do not view patients as broken, flawed, or immoral; rather, I see my patients as unique individuals who have imbalances that can be modified and corrected through holistic healing methods. And science — good, hard science — backs me up.

Who Can Benefit from This Book?

Anyone with any form of opioid dependency, regardless of the severity or scope of the dependency, can benefit from the natural therapies discussed in this book. These therapies will help you:

- Wean yourself off opioids

- Manage withdrawal symptoms

- Rebuild your health and vitality after withdrawal

- Manage chronic pain

What qualifies as dependency? You can be dependent on opioids because not taking them leaves you in debilitating pain. Or because you've been taking them, and when you stop, you don't feel well. Or because you don't function as well when you are not taking them. Or because you have uncontrollable intense cravings for opioids. Or because you are unable to stop taking opioids, even though using them is negatively affecting your personal relationships and finances. (Those last two are generally categorized as an *addiction* rather than a *dependency*, but the distinction can be a gray area.)

In general, someone who has been using opioids for a few weeks, while in recovery from an accident or surgery, is going to have a much easier time giving them up than the chronic addict who has been using them for years. But what constitutes dependency is different for different people.

Natural therapies are not a stand-alone strategy for quitting opioid use. Medical support and/or counseling is usually also necessary. If you have been prescribed opioids for short-term use, you will want to coordinate with your prescribing health-care provider to work out a schedule for weaning yourself off the medication. Those on the opposite end of the spectrum, suffering from chronic addiction, will require intensive medical support and/or counseling along with other local support.

If you still need medical support and counseling in order to kick the opioid habit, why would you also want to use natural therapies? As noted earlier, recidivism rates for opioid users are high. *Very* high. Withdrawal can be a grueling process, and many people fail. Natural therapies can lessen the physical symptoms, such as digestive issues and muscle spasms, but, more important, they can calm the mind so that patients do not feel as though they are "climbing out of their own skin," as many of my patients describe it. Moreover, natural healing modalities can address some of the more troubling symptoms of withdrawal that often thwart recovery, such as a deep sense of depression and loss of energy and spirit; these are, in fact, among the most common reasons for relapse.

Integrative Holistic Medicine

This book is designed to help you integrate and aggregate natural therapies with other efforts, leading to a better outcome in a shorter amount of time. I often focus on Traditional Chinese Medicine (TCM) because that is my training; I am a licensed doctor of acupuncture and Oriental medicine (DAOM). In my clinical practice, I have found both acupuncture and Chinese medicine to be very effective in treating opioid dependency. I have also found other natural healing modalities, like herbal medicine and mindfulness meditation, to be effective, and I integrate them into treatment protocols.

TCM is by nature a holistic system of healing. It views the body as a manifestation of energies and matter in which an imbalance in one area affects the entire system. Thus, addiction, disease, and pain conditions are simply patterns of imbalance. From this perspective, *imbalance*, not lack of willpower, is the cause of disease and addiction, and the job of the TCM practitioner is to help the patient regain balance. I think that most practitioners of any form of holistic medicine would agree.

TCM is a complex medical system, and it is easy for a practitioner to overexplain the subject and cause confusion. You cannot understand every detail and nuance of TCM without many years of study. However, a rudimentary knowledge of Chinese medicine will allow you to understand how it can benefit you and help you take responsibility for your health. I'll lay out the basic concepts in chapter 2, which will be helpful if you are unfamiliar with Chinese medicine. To take full advantage of all that Chinese medicine has to offer — and it is *very* effective in treating opioid dependency — I urge you to seek out a trained practitioner for guidance.

PART 1

Natural Therapies

to

COMBAT ADDICTION

CHAPTER 1

Opioid Dependency
A Breakdown

Opioid use and abuse in the United States has grown into a devastating epidemic. The U.S. Department of Health and Human Services (HHS) estimates that in 2016 more than 42,000 Americans died from overdosing on opioids.[4] That same year, more than 11.1 million Americans misused opioids, meaning that they took an opioid without a prescription or for a use other than what was prescribed; of that number, 2.1 million were categorized as having an "opioid use disorder" — that is, opioid dependency.[5] Those numbers represent exponential growth. In an analysis of its members, Blue Cross Blue Shield, one of the major health insurance companies in the United States, found that from 2010 to 2016 the number of people diagnosed with an addiction to opioids, including both legal prescription drugs like oxycodone and hydrocodone as well as illicit drugs like heroin, climbed by 493 percent.[6] And the statistics are getting worse.[7] In 2017, the HHS declared the opioid crisis to be a public health emergency.

The story line behind the unfolding disaster is well known. Opioids like oxycodone, hydrocodone, and methadone are prescription pain relievers. In the late 1990s, doctors, having been reassured by pharmaceutical manufacturers of the drugs' efficacy and safety, began prescribing opioids at an increasing pace to address their patients' acute and/or chronic pain. As we now know, the drugs are actually highly addictive. People who took them for prolonged periods found themselves suffering from intense addiction. They had a hard time managing their withdrawal, and often found it impossible.

In a knee-jerk reaction to the growing number of opioid addicts and deaths resulting from opioid overdosing, there has been a prohibitionist movement. Doctors are finding that they are restricted from prescribing opioids to pain patients or are simply choosing not to do so. As a result, we have a population of opioid refugees (patients who have been cut off from their legal opioid prescriptions) who must either suffer or seek alternative — and not always effective, advisable, or even legal — methods of pain relief.[8]

At the same time, the use of heroin (itself an opioid) is skyrocketing, not only as a result of the prescription opioid problem, but certainly worsened by it. The situation has become so critical that the U.S. Surgeon General recently released an advisory about it, urging healthcare providers and the family and friends of anyone with an opioid use disorder to keep nalaxone, an overdose-reversing drug, at hand.[9]

The opioid epidemic has left many caught up in a chaotic situation seeking relief from the torturous cycle of addiction. The story is complex, obviously, as politics, social dynamics, and medical pedagogy are among the factors that have shaped the ongoing crisis. However, those factors are beyond the scope of this book. Our focus is on helping people recover from opioid addiction. So let's take a look at how addiction works.

How Opioids Work

The human brain is programmed to use opioids. In fact, our own bodies produce opioids in the form of endorphins. The word *endorphin* is a blend of *endogenous* (growing within the body) and *morphine*. The brain and the pituitary gland produce endorphins in response to pain, stress, exercise, and pleasure, among other things. The endorphins circulate in our nervous system. They work like keys, and the locks into which they fit are opioid receptor sites in the brain. When activated by an endorphin key, an opioid receptor site signals the brain to release a controlled amount of dopamine, a neurotransmitter, which results in a sensation of pain relief and pleasure.

When it is functioning as it should, our body's natural endorphin-based opioid response system encourages us to seek out those things that bring pleasure — eating delicious food, exercising, having sex, laughing — and dampens sensations of pain.

Natural endorphins, however, can't hold a candle to the power of opioid drugs like methadone, oxycodone, fentanyl, and heroin. Opioid receptor sites do not discriminate between natural endorphins and these drugs; all opioids, no matter their source, act as keys to these locks. The drugs, however, stimulate a much stronger response. A flood of dopamine is released in the brain, with a resulting sensation of euphoria and powerful pain relief.

Because they are so incredibly effective at relieving pain, pharmaceutical opioids are valuable medications. The danger lies in their risk for causing addiction.

How Addiction Works

The brain can handle repeated overstimulation of its dopamine response for only a relatively short period. Eventually the receptor sites become less responsive to the opioid drugs. At first, increasing the drug dosage maintains the initial results, but with ongoing usage, the receptor sites become less and less reactive. At this point, the body's weaker endorphins cannot stimulate the release of dopamine in the way they did before the opioid drugs came into play. As a result, the opioid drug user has to continue to take opioids just to maintain emotional equilibrium and to function normally throughout the day.

The same sort of process can be seen in addictions to other substances, like alcohol and nicotine: addicts must take them in order to maintain emotional equilibrium and to function normally. But researchers are beginning to understand that opioids are especially addictive because they actually change the function and structure of the brain in a way that undermines our ability to resist them.[10] A 2002 study suggests that the widespread structural and functional effects of prescription opioids are likely to interfere with our normal decision-making processes and with our ability to abstain from opioids despite their known harmful potential.[11] We know, too, that the longer someone uses opioids, the more significant the impacts become.

Opioid addiction may also be linked to *conditioned association* — the memory that leads us to associate certain circumstances with drug use and the resulting feelings of pleasure. Opioids activate the brain's mesolimbic pathway, also called the reward pathway, which stimulates a dopamine release; the brain then creates a record or memory that associates the dopamine-induced good feelings with the environment in which they occur.[12] These memories lead drug abusers to crave drugs when they encounter those same circumstances, whether they be persons, places, or things, and they drive abusers to seek drugs despite the likely bad consequences; in fact, a 2007 study suggests that opioid dependency is a disease of learning and memory.[13]

Research into the mechanisms of dependency and addiction continues, but one thing is clear: opioids have an undeniable neurological impact, changing the actual physical structure of the brain and its processes.

Neuroplasticity: Rewiring the Brain

Until relatively recently, scientists believed that the brain developed in childhood and then remained static, or unchanged, during adulthood.[14] This implied that brain damage and degeneration were not reversible. However, modern research has shown that the brain has *neuroplasticity*, or the ability to develop new neural connections in order to circumvent damage and adapt to new input. In other words, the very structure of the brain can be changed.[15] What could possibly stimulate changes in the brain? Well, among other things, acupuncture can; it has been shown to enhance neuroplasticity and even to repair brain damage.[16] Meditation is another tool that, above and beyond all its other benefits, stimulates neuroplasticity.[17]

In their ability to stimulate neuroplasticity, practices like acupuncture and meditation offer a way to rewire neural networks to help people recover from opioid addiction, allowing them to circumvent or reverse the structural neurological changes induced by the drugs — and the addiction.

Recovery: Addressing Health Complications

Opioids are hard on the body, particularly when taken for a long time. People in recovery often face ongoing health complications, even months and years after withdrawal, ranging from low energy levels and poor sleep to digestive trouble, liver problems, cardiovascular issues, and poor memory and cognition. Such adverse effects on health can cause significant declines in quality of life and increases in health-care costs.[18]

In this area, natural therapies really shine. In addition to supporting the body through recovery, they restore and reinvigorate the body's organs and systems. We'll discuss the different protocols for addressing specific health conditions in chapter 10. Most of the protocols use an integrative approach, blending botanical, energetic, nutritional, and other strategies to bring the body back to balance.

CHAPTER 2

Chinese Medicine
Healing Body, Mind, and Spirit

We are learning that planet Earth can take only so much abuse, neglect, and toxic buildup before the natural ecological balance is disrupted. This same principle holds true for our health: the body can compensate for imbalances for only so long before a critical point is reached and it can no longer cope. Opioid use can be likened to a huge dump of poisonous chemicals into a river: not only are the negative results immediate, but bringing the river back to a healthy ecosystem may take years or even decades. Each individual part of the ecosystem must be restored before the river is healthy again.

TCM has always viewed the universe as a macrocosm and our body as a microcosm that mimics the universe. In TCM, the body cannot be separated from the mind and spirit. Wellness is not simply a matter of being disease-free; rather, wellness requires a thriving body, a clear mind, and a peaceful spirit. From this perspective, to overcome opioid dependency, the body, mind, and spirit must become unified in balance.

An Overview

The origins of TCM are shrouded in mystery and myth; all we know for sure is that it dates back to before the time of writing. Originally practiced by priest-doctors known as shamans, who used primitive tools such as stones, TCM has developed into a well-documented, evidence-based system of medicine with important modern-day applications.

It is important to note that many theories of Chinese medicine have developed over the centuries, and practitioners agree on no single dogma. Rather, TCM has developed as a subtle and complex treatment modality whose wide-ranging applications have been repeatedly proven powerful and effective by scientific research.

Chinese medicine began developing a keen interest in opioid addiction treatment about 200 years ago. At that time, Western countries trading with China had developed concerning trade deficits, as they did not produce many commodities that China required. England resolved this dilemma by developing a drug trade targeting China, shipping in opium from India and other poppy-growing regions. While this would seem unconscionable today, at the time the West saw it as good economics and did not give much weight to the ethical implications. Realizing the detrimental effects of opium on its society, China pushed back, and the two historic Opium Wars of 1839 and 1856 resulted. While the true circumstances and motivations for those wars are argued to this day, the one fact that no one disputes is that these wars permanently altered the course of China's history. (As often happens, present-day circumstances have an eerie similarity to historical events. Currently, the United States is experiencing the dire economic and social impacts of opioid addiction. In a reversal of roles, Chinese drug traffickers are the ones bringing opium to the West; several are under indictment by the U.S. Department of Justice on charges of manufacturing the highly addictive opioid drug fentanyl, selling it over the Internet, and shipping the contraband to the West by international postal services.)

In any case, the Chinese in the nineteenth century had powerful motivation for developing treatment strategies for opioid addiction, and they did so very effectively. Modern clinical studies show that TCM now has a wide spectrum of positive effects; as one group of researchers from the Chinese National Institute on Drug Dependence noted in 2006:

> There are some advantages in using TCM for opiate detoxification, including less harmful side effects, high safety and ideal effects in the inhibition of protracted withdrawal symptoms and relapse. Co-administration of TCM with modern medicine shows some synergistic effects in detoxification. Many TCM for detoxification also have efficacy in the rehabilitation of abnormal body functions induced by chronic drug use, including improving immune function, increasing working memory and preventing neurological disorder. Given that TCM is effective in the prevention of relapse and causes fewer side effects, it may be used widely in the treatment of opiate addiction.[19]

Chinese versus Western Medicine

Modern Western medicine consistently produces miraculous healing feats through heroic high-tech interventions. This leaves us to question how an ancient, low-impact, low-tech medical system could play any relevant role in something as serious as the opioid epidemic or, for that matter, any modern health concerns. To understand the value of integrating TCM into our health-care system, it is important to describe the areas in which a subtle healing art such as TCM can complement and augment modern medicine. Here are a few examples of ways in which modern medicine and TCM collaborate for better patient outcomes.

Case Studies

If someone were to experience a car accident that resulted in traumatic injury, like a broken leg or punctured lung, he would be wise to get himself whisked straight to an emergency room rather than an acupuncturist's office. However, in the days and weeks after that emergency treatment, he could turn to acupuncture and herbal medicine to speed up his recovery process, address his pain, and shorten the duration of the pain medications he might have to take.

If someone were diagnosed with stage 3 pancreatic cancer, she would be wise to explore the possibilities of gene therapy and other emerging treatment modalities rather than simply drinking a cup of herbal tea. Yet major cancer centers throughout the country employ licensed acupuncturists who work to bring the cancer patient's body back into balance and lessen the chances of recurrence following treatment. Additionally, acupuncture is highly advocated to treat nausea during chemotherapy.

If a child has cerebral palsy, acupuncture and herbs are not likely to reverse the condition. Nevertheless, acupuncture and herbal therapy can help improve the child's motor function so that the child's mobility improves. Additionally, acupuncture can help with digestion, spasms, and drooling. While acupuncture cannot cure cerebral palsy, it can drastically improve the quality of life for a child with this disease.

If you have developed type 2 diabetes and are insulin dependent, it is improbable that acupuncture and herbs are going to reverse your condition, but they can help you moderate your blood-sugar levels so that less cellular damage occurs. Moreover, if you are prediabetic or insulin resistant, acupuncture, herbs, and lifestyle adjustments can fully resolve the issue before it has a chance to develop into full-blown diabetes.

Western medicine struggles in finding effective protocols that reverse chronic disease, eliminate pain, or cure addiction; these are the areas in which TCM shines. TCM is not appropriate for critical care; this is the area in which modern medicine excels. When looked at in this light, it is clear that the two healing modalities are perfect bedfellows.

Energies, Elements, and Fundamental Substances

Much of TCM has its foundation in Taoist beliefs. The Tao is an ancient text written by Lao-tzu, a philosopher of the sixth century B.C.E., describing how humans can live in harmony with nature to preserve health and happiness. It teaches that we can achieve a fortunate life only by maintaining lifestyle practices that promote balance: physical wellness, emotional equilibrium, and cultural peace. In line with that philosophy, the subtle yet profound effects of Chinese medicine work to bring balance to all the energies and substances that flow through and harmonize the body, mind, and spirit.

Yin and Yang

Yin and yang are two opposing yet complementary forces of the universe and everything in it, including the body. Each must be balanced relative to the other to ensure good health and vitality.

In terms of the body, yin is generally thought of as substance, and yang as energy. Yin is to yang like a log is to a fire: we must nourish yin so that our yang energy can burn long and bright. Yang makes things happen; yin provides the material necessary for things to happen.

In the body, yin is matter like blood, fluids, and tissues, while yang is energy and heat. Yin is cold, damp, and feminine; yang is hot, dry, and masculine. But there is no absolute yin or yang. As the yin-yang symbol shows us, every yin manifestation contains a bit of yang, and every yang manifestation contains a bit of yin. And these qualities manifest only as comparisons. For example, warm liquid is yang compared to cold liquid, but warm liquid is yin compared to hot liquid.

The inseparable forces of yin and yang are in constant negotiation, balancing against each other. They do not permit homeostasis but are constantly flowing and changing. In this way, they animate the human body.

All disease patterns pass through phases of yin and yang until they are resolved. If you sprain your ankle, at first it is yang: hot and inflamed. As this yang condition transforms to yin, the swelling goes down and the ankle becomes cold and stiff. Ideally, a balance of energies is eventually reached and the ankle is healed.

An opioid dependency often initiates a yin deficiency. Stress consumes yin in the body, and opioid use places physical stress on the body, and often emotional stress too (hiding a dependency can be stressful, as can trying to overcome the dependency). Without yin,

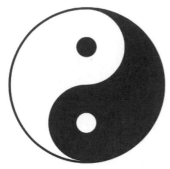

Yin is cold, damp, and feminine.
Yang is hot, dry, and masculine.
These forces are constantly in flow,
balancing against each other.

yang suffers as well; continuing the previous metaphor, there is no log to feed the fire. Thus yang deficiency eventually results. Thus yin and yang deficiencies are common diagnoses for people recovering from opioid dependency. In order for them to fully heal, these energies must be revived and brought into balance.

Qi (Vital Energy)

Qi, pronounced "chee" and sometimes spelled *chi or ch'i*, is our vital energy. Qi is the source of all movement in the body: fluids, energy, and matter ascending, descending, entering, and leaving. It circulates throughout the body following prescribed pathways, called channels or meridians.

Qi protects the body against external and internal pathogenic factors. When qi is insufficient or stagnant, the body declines and disease can develop. The goal of Chinese medicine is to ensure that qi is able to move freely, that it is moving in the correct direction, and that there is an abundance of it in the body.

We acquire qi through the food, liquids, and air that we consume. Certain herbs can stimulate it as well. We can manipulate qi flow in the body through acupuncture, which stimulates points on the meridians.

People who use opioid drugs for a long time typically do not eat well and do not treat their body well. As a result, qi production diminishes; qi deficiency is a common TCM diagnosis with those recovering from opioid dependency.

Jing (Essence)

Essence, known as *jing*, is that aspect of the body that is the basis for all growth, development, and sexuality. Prenatal essence (sometimes called congenital essence) is that part of the body's essence we inherit from our parents. Postnatal essence, which is akin to an inborn constitution, determines each of our growth patterns.

We are born with a finite amount of prenatal essence. It can never be replaced if it is lost, but it can be supplemented by acquired essence, which is derived from food and herbs. Proper lifestyle habits, such as sound sleep at night, help preserve essence.

If we do not cultivate qi properly, our body is forced to dip into its reserves of essence for the energy it needs. Unfortunately, people who use opioids on a regular basis generally do not eat well, sleep well, or practice any of the proper lifestyle habits necessary to maintain essence. As a result, they suffer from depleted essence, or what Western natural health advocates often refer to as adrenal fatigue or adrenal exhaustion. This is a common condition seen in opioid recovery, with indications of severe exhaustion that does not abate quickly.

Shen (Spirit)

The spirit, or *shen*, represents the forces that shape our personality, including psycho-emotional aspects. This is not the spirit of religious traditions; rather, it is our inner light. The heart houses shen, and it can be observed by trained practitioners through a certain brightness of the eyes. Shen disturbances generally refer to mental disorders.

Blood

Blood is a fundamental substance in the body that nourishes and moistens the whole organism. The body is dependent on a high quality and abundance of nourishing blood to maintain elastic skin, vibrant eyes, and healthy organs. Blood and qi are interdependent: qi moves blood, and blood nourishes qi production. When either is deficient, disharmony occurs, leading to ill health.

ACTUALLY, THERE IS NO SUCH THING AS BLOOD STAGNATION

Much is lost in translation in Chinese medicine. The term *blood stagnation* was taken from the Chinese *xue yu*, which is more accurately translated as "blood silt disease." Silt is defined as fine sand, clay, or other rock particles carried by running water and deposited as sediment, especially in a channel or river. You can imagine a patient's confusion when an acupuncturist explains that she has blood silt; she may ask how silt got into her blood. Instead, the diagnosis is meant to refer to blood that is less than optimal and therefore sluggish or impeded by cellular waste in the circulation system. Rather than trying to explain all of this to patients, practitioners took to using the term *blood stagnation*, which is easier for Westerners to understand.

People recovering from opioid addiction often suffer from blood deficiency, indicated by lusterless skin, fatigue, vision problems, cold hands and feet, and so on. They also often suffer from blood stagnation, which happens when blood flow is sluggish or impeded and can cause sharp or stabbing pain, a purplish complexion and tongue, and numbness in the extremities.

The Five Elements

The five elements — Water, Wood, Fire, Earth, and Metal — are the different aspects of qi, and together they make up the foundational energies of the natural world. Like yin and yang, the five elements are interdependent, and they rise and fall in cycles of relationship to each other.

- *The cycle of elements:* Water nourishes Wood, Wood fuels Fire, Fire makes Earth (ashes), Earth yields Metal, Metal produces Water (condensation).

- *The cycle of life:* Birth (Water) is followed by growth (Wood), maturation (Fire), reflection (Metal), and death (Water).

- *The cycle of the seasons:* The first is winter (Water); then comes spring (Wood), summer (Fire), late summer (Earth), fall (Metal), and then back to winter (Water).

- *The cycle of influence:* Water can extinguish Fire, Fire can melt Metal, Metal can cut Wood, Wood can contain Earth, and Earth can absorb Water.

The body is a microcosm of the natural world, and so these same elements and cycles are also at work within us. When the elements within us are out of balance with one another, the cycles are thrown out of balance, and disruption or disease results. If we know how to influence the elemental energies within us — and acupuncture, herbs, nutrition, meditation, and other aspects of holistic medicine do just that — we can influence the cycles within us and so bring the body back into balance. And indeed, in chapter 7 you'll find protocols for treating opioid dependency by correcting elemental imbalances.

THE FIVE ELEMENTS: CORRELATIONS

ELEMENT	ORGAN	COLOR	EMOTION
Water	Kidneys	Blue	Fear
Wood	Liver	Green	Anger
Fire	Heart	Red	Lack of joy
Earth	Spleen	Yellow	Worry
Metal	Lungs	White	Grief

FIVE ELEMENT MEDITATION

As shown in the chart on page 27, each of the five elements correlates to a particular organ, color, and emotion. The Five Element Meditation can be a powerful tool for activating resonances among the energies of the elements, organs, colors, and emotions, thereby helping to heal, tonify, and balance all of them.

You will need to know the approximate shape and location of the organs for this meditation. If necessary, take the time for a little research before beginning.

Begin by sitting or standing in a comfortable position. Close your eyes. Breathe deeply through your nose.

Visualize your lungs. Breathe clean white light deeply into your lungs (belly breathing). Fill your lungs with the light. Exhale murky white light, releasing any grief. Continue for several minutes.

Next, visualize your kidneys. Begin to breathe brilliant blue light into your kidneys. Fill your kidneys with the light. Exhale murky blue breath, releasing any fear. Continue for several minutes.

Now visualize your liver, and begin to breathe brilliant green light into it. Fill your liver with the light. Exhale murky green breath, releasing any anger. Continue for several minutes.

Moving on, visualize your heart, and begin to breathe brilliant red light into it. Fill your heart with the light. Exhale murky red breath, releasing any sadness. Continue for several minutes.

Finally, visualize your spleen, and begin to breathe brilliant yellow light into it. Fill your spleen with the light. Exhale murky yellow breath, releasing any worry. Continue for several minutes.

Organ Systems of TCM

The concept of the organs in TCM is radically different from that of contemporary Western medicine. Understanding this difference is crucial, because the physiology and pathology of the organs are fundamental to understanding and treating disease. Chinese medical theory is not a quick study, but let's break it down to the basics here. (Note: Throughout this book, TCM organ systems are capitalized to distinguish them from the Western conceptualizations.)

To begin, in TCM, an *organ* is actually a system, not a structure. Each organ system includes not only the physical organ, as understood in Western medicine, but also an array of interrelated functions and the channel that carries the energy of that system. For example, in Western medicine, the kidneys are organs that collect and excrete urine. In Chinese medicine, the Kidneys comprise the physical kidney organs and the Kidney channel (the energetic pathway of Kidney qi), and they are a storehouse of jing, the center of yin and yang, and the controller of the body's waterways, among other things.

Chinese medicine even recognizes some organ systems that have no parallel in Western medicine, like the San Jiao (Triple Burner), an organ system responsible for metabolism.

All the organ systems can be divided into yin and yang categories:

- *The yin organs* are the Kidneys, Liver, Heart (Pericardium), Spleen, and Lungs. They are considered to be relatively deep in the body and generally more solid, and they are involved with the regulation, manufacture, and storage of fundamental substances such as blood and essence.

- *The yang organs* are the Stomach, Gallbladder, Large Intestine, Small Intestine, Bladder, and San Jiao. They are generally hollow and considered to be closer to the surface or exterior of the body. They do not store substances but are instead involved with ongoing processes of exchange, receiving, separating, distributing, and excreting substances.

Each organ system has an impact on the other organ systems when it becomes imbalanced; additionally, each organ has an impact on the emotions. Chinese medicine views each person as a holistic interactive entity rather than a collection of individual parts and pieces. This is how Chinese medicine is able to differentiate disease patterns and devise effective treatment strategies. One disease can have many different patterns depending on a person's individual physiology, genetic dispositions, and lifestyle habits.

In this book, we focus primarily on the five organ systems that correlate to the five elements, because identifying and correcting elemental imbalances is a powerful method for treating opioid dependency and facilitating recovery. Let's take a closer look.

SYMPTOMS AND IMBALANCES

In describing patterns of imbalance for the organs, I list the indications, or symptoms, that generally manifest with those imbalances. Note that an imbalance will not necessarily result in every indication that is listed. For a diagnosis, you would look for a number of those indications to begin to develop, thereby manifesting a *pattern* of imbalance.

Kidneys: Water Element

Among other things, the Kidneys are the base of all yin and yang in the body. They control the waterways and regulate fluid balance in the body, store jing (essence), and produce marrow, which is essential for the formation of bone, the spinal cord, blood, and the brain.

The Kidneys correlate to the ears (they are said to "open into the ears") and influence hearing. They also manifest in the hair; vital, lush, shiny hair is a sign of good Kidney health.

In people suffering from opioid dependency, two common Kidney imbalances are Kidney yin deficiency (see page 142) and Kidney yang deficiency (see page 144). While it's true that opioid use contributes to Kidney deficiency, it may also be true that many people who are prescribed opioids have preexisting Kidney defiency. Chronic lower back pain, for example, a symptom of Kidney deficiency, is a common diagnosis for people who are prescribed opioids.[20]

COMMON SYMPTOMS OF KIDNEY IMBALANCES

- Afternoon and night sweats
- Low energy
- Knee pain and weakness
- Chronic lower back pain and weakness
- Fear and phobias
- Anxiety and panic attacks
- Ringing in the ears or hearing loss
- Premature aging, including graying of the hair
- Memory loss
- Sexual dysfunctions, including impotence
- Infertility
- Urinary disorders

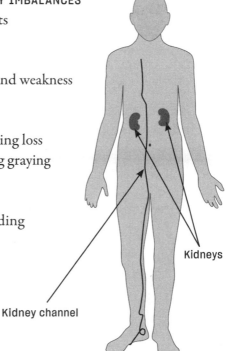

Kidneys

Kidney channel

Liver: Wood Element

The Liver spreads the qi of all the organs in all directions, governing the free flow of qi that is necessary for the healthy function of the body. It controls the tendons and joints, providing them with nourishing blood, and correlates to the eyes (it is said to "open into the eyes").

Since pain is a symptom of qi stagnation, Liver imbalances that cause qi stagnation anywhere in the body can contribute to pain syndromes. According to TCM, any pain in the joints indicates a Liver imbalance.

In people suffering from opioid dependency, Liver qi stagnation (see page 149) is common.

COMMON SYMPTOMS OF LIVER IMBALANCES
- Headaches
- Premenstrual syndrome (PMS)
- Anger and frustration
- Acid reflux
- Irritable bowel syndrome (IBS)
- Joint pain
- Osteoarthritis and stiff joints
- Brittle nails
- Lack of vision and direction in planning one's life

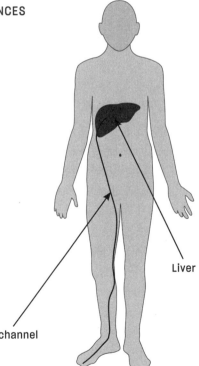

Liver

Liver channel

Heart: Fire Element

Many societies through the ages have associated the Heart with love, as does TCM. In fact, TCM theory holds that the Heart governs all emotions, and a healthy Heart enables emotional and sexual warmth as well as the ability to feel joy. TCM also holds that the Heart controls the blood vessels, which more closely aligns with the Western medicinal model.

In people suffering from opioid dependency, a common Heart imbalance is blood and qi deficiency resulting in impaired cognition (see page 155).

COMMON SYMPTOMS OF HEART IMBALANCES

- Emotional instability
- Insomnia
- Pain and burning sensation on the tongue
- Palpitations
- Heart disease
- Poor memory
- Mouth and tongue ulcers

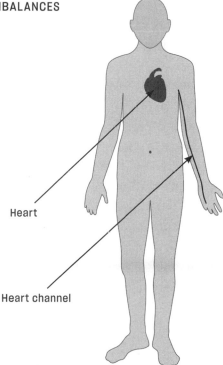

Heart

Heart channel

Spleen: Earth Element

TCM's perspective on the Spleen energetic organ system does not closely align with Western medicine's understanding of spleen and its functional aspects. According to TCM, the Spleen transforms and transports foods and fluids, making it central to digestion and nutritional absorption. If the Spleen does not manage fluids effectively, they can accumulate in the body, causing pain and a feeling of heaviness.

The Spleen controls the body's "upright qi" — the power of qi to counteract gravity and hold the organs in place, preventing prolapses. It also manufactures blood, and Spleen qi keeps the blood in the vessels. Easy bruising — that is, blood spilling out from the vessels — is a diagnostic sign of Spleen qi deficiency.

In people suffering from opioid dependency, Spleen qi deficiency (see page 160) is a common Spleen imbalance.

COMMON SYMPTOMS OF SPLEEN IMBALANCES

- Poor appetite
- Gas and abdominal distension
- Stomach pain
- Dampness or phlegm
- Pain that worsens in wet conditions and humidity
- Achy pain syndromes with a feeling of heaviness
- Tiredness or weakness
- Loose stools
- Prolapsed organs
- Uterine bleeding
- Varicose veins
- Easy bruising
- Obsessive worry
- Lack of empathy

Spleen

Spleen channel

Lungs: Metal Element

The Lungs are said to "open into the nose," and this energetic organ system includes the sinuses. It is closely related to the immune system and is central in defending the body from pathogenic invasions, like viral colds and influenza. The Lung system also correlates to the skin, and an imbalance in this system may be indicated by skin sensitivity.

In people suffering from opioid dependency, a common Lung imbalance is Lung qi deficiency (see page 166).

COMMON SYMPTOMS OF LUNG IMBALANCES

- Coughing
- Bronchitis, asthma
- Chronic obstructive pulmonary disease (COPD)
- Gentle touch feels painful
- Sinusitis
- Frequent colds or flu
- Sadness or unresolved grief
- Dogmatism
- Lack of self-worth
- Poor boundaries

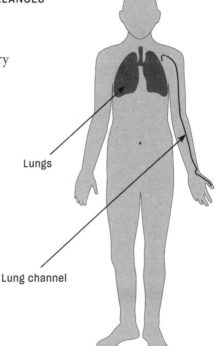

Lungs

Lung channel

Causes of Disease in TCM

There is an understanding in Chinese medicine that wellness is a natural state and illness is the result of any number of pathogenic influences, emotional stressors, or poor lifestyle habits. When the body is in harmony or balance, it is able to resist pathogens and will not develop chronic diseases that can lead to premature aging and degeneration. Wellness in Chinese medicine does not simply refer to an absence of disease; rather, a healthy person is happy, healthy, and pain-free. In an effort to understand how to obtain wellness, we must first explore how a person can develop disease and imbalance.

Six Pathogenic Factors

From the perspective of TCM, everything in the universe is interconnected. Any changes in the universe, such as changes in the weather, influence humans. Weather is characterized by six energies that can cause disharmony in the body. The Six Pathogenic Factors, as they are known, are generally opportunistic; they cause disease only when our immune system is weakened.

- *Wind* causes symptoms that wander and change.

- *Cold* causes the sudden onset of symptoms of chilliness, headache, and body aches.

- *Damp* causes sluggishness, lethargy, and sticky discharges.

- *Heat* (sometimes called fire) causes fever, inflammation, constipation, and dry skin.

- *Dryness* is closely related to heat but involves more drying of bodily fluids. Symptoms include dry eyes, dry nose, dry mouth, and dry cough.

- *Toxins* are virulent pathogens that are not associated with climactic factors and can attack even the normally resistant individual.

INTERNAL WIND

Internal wind is one of the more difficult Chinese medical concepts to explain in plain language. External wind relates to external pathogens like viruses. Internal wind arises from internal imbalances. It is most often associated with imbalances of the Liver and the Wood element. Internal wind commonly develops in the elderly as their bodies become more frail and deficient but can develop at any age.

Symptoms of Internal Wind

- Sudden onset of disease

- Pain that moves around

- Muscle spasms and cramps

- Arthritis that moves from joint to joint

- Sudden onset of headache or migraine with vertigo

- Tremors, spasms, and shaking

- Dizziness or vertigo

- Rashes that appear suddenly

- Itchy skin conditions

- Stroke

- Rigid limbs or paralysis

- Parkinson's disease

Genetic Factors

Chinese medicine has recognized the influence of familial disease patterns for thousands of years, and practitioners have inquired about family history long before DNA was discovered. Some people are under the false perception that genetic imbalances cannot be positively influenced. Just as a change in diet and exercise can improve the prognosis for someone whose parent has had a heart attack, Chinese tonic herbs and other medical techniques can improve the prognosis for all types of genetically related diseases.

Poor Diet

Improper eating habits can cause imbalances in many organ systems. Good eating habits are generally well understood in our culture, with wellness having become a popular topic in the media. Organic whole foods are always a good idea. Chinese medicine would advise against any excesses such as too much salt, which would damage Kidneys; too many spicy foods, which may damage the Lungs; or excessive amounts of iced drinks or raw foods, which can cause dampness and damage the Spleen.

Poor Exercise Habits

Proper exercise is important in keeping blood and qi flowing. Brisk walking, qi gong, tai qi, and yoga are the preferred types of exercise in Chinese medicine. Vigorous exercise or very hard physical work can cause imbalances and should be avoided.

Poor Sleep

Having sound sleep during the night is a vital part of maintaining wellness in Chinese medicine. Broken sleep patterns, wakefulness at night, and prolonged sleep deprivation are all reason for concern.

Emotional Factors

In TCM theory, one of the major causes of disease is emotion, whether negative (e.g., anger, worry, fear, fright, anxiety, grief) or positive (e.g., joy). All of these emotions are normal, and everyone experiences them at different times. Emotional responses can cause disease and injure the vital organs if they are out of proportion to the situation or if they are chronic. Alternatively, if an organ system becomes deficient or out of balance, the related emotions can occur chronically. It is often a chicken-or-egg question: Did a bodily imbalance cause an abnormal emotional response, or did the emotions damage the organ system? All of the emotions originate in the Heart, and serious emotional disorders are considered to be disorders of Heart shen.

As we've discussed, in Chinese medicine, emotional wellness is as important to vitality and health as physical wellness. While it is well established that opioid use leads to physical deterioration, the relationship between opioid use and emotional/psychological health is less certain. Chronic opioid users have a higher-than-average rate of psychological and emotional issues, but whether those issues contribute to opioid dependency or are caused by it is still unknown. In fact, both may be true.

One 2010 study, an assessment of more than 1,000 recovering heroin addicts, concluded:

> Addiction is a relapsing chronic condition in which psychiatric phenomena play a crucial role. . . . The hypothesis that mood, anxiety and impulse-control dysregulation [are] at the very core both of the origins and the clinical phenomenology of addiction should be considered, as well as the crucial role played by psychiatric manifestations as addiction progresses.[21]

The study found that the participants could be divided into five groups based on their dominant emotional imbalances. Interestingly, the psychological profiles for those five groups aligned with the personality types of the five elements of Chinese medicine (Water, Wood, Earth, Fire, Metal). Practitioners of Chinese medicine have long worked with the five elements to reinforce emotional balance and psychological wellness in their patients. Because psychological influences have such a strong connection to opioid dependency, the five elements offer us a way to treat the addiction on a psychological level. Let's take a closer look at each element in relation to the 2010 study.

Panic/Anxiety: Water Element

Of the study's participants, 22.3 percent reported dominant feelings of panic and anxiety such as "fear of travelling by bus, train or subway," panic attacks with nausea and light-headedness, and social anxiety. For this group, the study's authors noted, "Generalised fear is a feature, with the need to avoid certain things, places or activities in order to prevent panicking." These are all classic symptoms of Kidney deficiency and a Water element imbalance.

Violence/Suicide: Wood Element

A group comprising 19.7 percent of the study's participants displayed violent outbursts with destructive aspects and physical aggression. Sometimes that anger turned inward, resulting in suicidal tendencies. As the authors noted, this group "longs for death." These characteristics describe Wood influences, as this element correlates with the emotion of anger. The Liver is the yin organ of the Wood element, and this group displayed additional symptoms of Liver qi stagnation, such as restlessness and feeling upset much of the time.

Sensitivity/Psychoticism: Fire Element

This group, which comprised 19.4 percent of the study's participants, had psychotic factors ranging toward extreme paranoia. They "have the impression that others stare at them or speak about them, may do something against them, . . . do not sympathise with them or approve of their behaviour. . . . These behaviours may be defined as psychotic as long as the patient is convinced that others control or influence their thoughts, in some cases actually being identified as imposed from out-side that individual's mind." In TCM, this is a disorder of Heart shen. The Heart is the yin organ of the Fire element, and it is said to house the mind and all emotions.

Worthlessness/Feeling Trapped: Earth Element

This group, which comprised 14.2 percent of the study's participants, was dominated by feelings of worthlessness and being trapped, marked by obsessive-compulsive behaviors, worrying, and an inability to concentrate. In TCM, the *yi* (intellect) is said to reside in the Spleen, which is the yin organ of the Earth element. An overriding theme in patients with Earth element imbalances is the feeling "No one cares about me," which develops into a sense of worthlessness. Obsessive thoughts and behaviors are classic symptoms of Earth element imbalances. Additionally, the Spleen controls water metabolism in the body. When the Spleen is not functioning optimally, internal dampness begins to accumulate; mentally, this would manifest as a feeling of foggy-headedness, with difficulty concentrating.

Somatization: Metal Element

This group, comprising 24.4 percent of the study's participants, had dominant characterizations of somatization, or the manifestation of physical complaints without medical cause, sometimes resulting from the conversion of mental symptoms to physical ones. Somatization is often a feature of opioid withdrawal. These participants reported, among other things, feelings of breathlessness and chest pain, which are classic symptoms of a Metal element imbalance. The Lungs are the yin organs of the Metal element. Qi flow to the Lungs is most active between 3:00 and 5:00 a.m., according to TCM, and participants in this group reported that they "wake up early at dawn and cannot get back to sleep" — a specific symptom of imbalance of the Metal element. This group also experienced heightened interpersonal sensitivity; the Metal element establishes our personal boundaries, and those with Metal element imbalances can be hypersensitive to others getting in their personal space, literally or figuratively.

What to Expect from a TCM Practitioner

TCM has five primary branches of practice: acupuncture, herbal medicine, *tui na* (therapeutic massage), medical qi gong (energy healing), and nutritional therapy. A TCM practitioner will be a licensed acupuncturist (L.Ac.); the L.Ac. accreditation means that the practitioner has received a 4-year postgraduate degree (3 years if their school did not train in Chinese herbalism) and passed a national board exam through the National Certification Commission for Acupuncture and Oriental Medicine (or an equivalent state exam). Those with DAOM credentials (Doctor of Acupuncture and Oriental Medicine) have, in addition to all that, another 2 years of study at the doctorate level of training in Oriental medicine.

Your practitioner will ask you to fill out a wide-ranging questionnaire and ask you a number of questions relating to your health and symptoms. He or she may also examine your tongue, take your pulses, and palpate areas for tenderness.

Many patients new to acupuncture are nervous about the treatment. There is no need for worry. Licensed acupuncturists are highly skilled. The needles are hair thin. They typically cause no pain, though you may feel a slight pinch when they are inserted. The needles usually stay in place for 20 to 30 minutes while you relax, and then the practitioner will gently remove them.

Your practitioner may utilize tui na massage or medical qi gong healing techniques during your treatment. He or she may give dietary recommendations or herbal prescriptions as part of your healing plan. Other practices are also often prescribed in treatment, including moxibustion (see page 48), Taoist meditations, and tai chi exercises.

As you'll learn in chapter 3, acupuncture and other TCM healing techniques are generally not single-session cures. Your practitioner will work with you to set up a schedule for ongoing treatments that will work, over time, to bring your body and all its energies into balance.

Acupuncture and Acupressure
Clearing Blockages and Stagnation

Acupuncture involves inserting hair-thin needles at specific points on the body, called acupoints, to stimulate the meridians and the energy they carry. Stimulation of acupoints helps move qi, resolve stagnation, and balance the body and its systems. Acupuncture is widely used to relieve pain and to treat various physical, mental, and emotional conditions.

Acupressure is similar to acupuncture except that it uses finger pressure, rather than needles, on acupoints. Acupressure is considered to be less powerful than acupuncture, but it can be used effectively at home as part of a self-care regimen to promote healing, reduce stress, and alleviate fatigue.

Acupuncture can be a powerful therapy in our nation's battle against opioid dependency. To begin, studies from around the world have proven that acupuncture is an effective alternative to opioids in pain management; if pain patients can be prescribed acupuncture instead of opioids, we entirely circumvent the risk of dependency. For people who are trying to overcome a dependency, acupuncture has been shown to reduce cravings for opioids and to modulate or even eliminate some of the uncomfortable symptoms experienced during withdrawal. After withdrawal, we can turn to acupuncture to restore health to the whole body, including neural networks in the brain, and we can target the treatments to help heal particular organ systems, elemental imbalances, qi blockages, and so forth.

Pain Management

In the face of a national opioid epidemic, medical systems in the United States are looking more and more to nonpharmacologic strategies for pain. Numerous federal regulatory agencies have advised or mandated that health-care systems and providers offer drug-free treatment options for pain, including acupuncture, physical therapy, spinal cord manipulation, yoga, tai chi, and cognitive behavioral therapy. Among these, acupuncture stands out as the most specific in targeting the endorphin neurosystem that mediates the pain response.[22]

In the spring of 2017, the U.S. Food and Drug Administration (FDA) released a guide, called the "FDA Blueprint for Prescriber Education for Extended-Release and Long-Acting Opioid Analgesics," that recommended doctors become informed about nonpharmacologic options for pain control to help avoid the overuse of opioids. Thereafter, a joint commission made up of members from the National Academies of Science, Engineering, and Medicine formed at the FDA's request to assess the abuse and misuse of opioid medications. The resulting report systematically summarized the evidence for acupuncture's clinical benefits in treating pain. The commission's research resulted in a mandate for hospitals to provide nonpharmacologic pain management treatment modalities such as acupuncture by July 2018.[23]

Acupuncture is now being recognized as a first-line treatment for pain, before opiates are prescribed, to avoid the development of opioid addiction. It is being implemented in hospital settings as diverse as surgery recovery, stroke rehabilitation, and pain clinics to treat a variety of pain and mobility issues. It has even been found to be useful in the emergency room; a randomized trial of acupuncture versus morphine to treat emergency department patients with acute pain concluded that acupuncture worked better and faster than morphine, with far fewer side effects.[24]

Acupuncture has also been shown to be an effective adjunctive analgesic for postsurgical treatment, reducing the use of opioids across a wide range of both minor and major surgical procedures.[25] Some studies have reported that acupuncture can reduce the consumption of opioid-like medication by more than 60 percent following surgery.[26]

Low back pain is one of the most common reasons why people seek help from their doctor.[27] A comprehensive review of studies on nonpharmacologic pain-reduction treatment modalities found that acupuncture is one of the most effective for this kind of pain, and in early 2017, the American College of Physicians published guidelines for the treatment of low back pain strongly suggesting the use of acupuncture, multidisciplinary rehabilitation, mindfulness-based stress reduction, tai chi, yoga, and so on.[28]

When the U.S. Department of Veterans Affairs and branches of the U.S. military began using acupuncture for pain and stress management, the use of opiates and other pain medications among personnel decreased dramatically. Opioid prescriptions decreased by 45 percent, muscle relaxants by 34 percent, nonsteroidal anti-inflammatory drugs (NSAIDs) by 42 percent, and benzodiazepines by 14 percent.[29] As a result, the military is rapidly incorporating acupuncture into its treatments for service members.[30]

In the context of this book, it would be impossible to notate the hundreds of studies that have been performed demonstrating acupuncture's efficacy in treating pain syndromes. It has been found to be effective in relieving pain for a wide range of conditions that includes osteoarthritis, allergic rhinitis, chemotherapy-induced nausea and vomiting, chronic lower back pain, headaches and migraines, postoperative pain, and many more.[31] I've cited just a handful of the most relevant studies here; you can find many more online via the National Institutes of Health's PubMed database.

Acupuncture for Addiction and Withdrawal

As far back as 1996, the World Health Organization (WHO) accepted acupuncture as a therapy for drug addiction. The U.S. National Institutes of Health (NIH) accepted acupuncture as an integrative therapy for addiction in 1997;[32] more recently, a detailed research review concluded that acupuncture is a viable treatment option for opioid addiction.[33]

Acupuncture is an effective treatment for opioid addiction because it stimulates the same endorphin cycle that opioids do, thereby minimizing cravings for the drugs, and it also eases withdrawal symptoms. Those symptoms can vary in intensity depending on the intensity of the addiction and the rate of withdrawal. Someone who abruptly halts an opioid habit, for example, will experience rapid detox and potentially severe withdrawal symptoms. Stepping down slowly by reducing opioid use gradually is generally a less intense process.

Whether a person is going through rapid detox or a gradual cessation, acupuncture can be highly effective in ameliorating physical symptoms. It works to normalize the digestive system, avoiding the nausea, vomiting, abdominal cramping, and diarrhea associated with withdrawal, and it lessens muscle cramping, spasms, and achiness. It also reduces cravings, soothes the nerves and emotions, and promotes good sleep. In this way, it helps the patient through the withdrawal process and minimizes the chances of relapse.

Study of acupuncture's mechanism of action during withdrawal is ongoing, and many questions remain. Nevertheless, it's known that acupuncture has a direct impact on the brain by activating the body's endogenous opioids and opioid-receptor sites. One study noted, "Neurochemical and behavioral evidence have shown that acupuncture helps reduce the effects of positive and negative reinforcement involved in opiate addiction by modulating mesolimbic dopamine neurons."[34] Research with rats has shown that acupuncture ameliorates the symptoms of morphine withdrawal.[35] And auricular acupuncture (acupuncture of the ear) has been shown to evoke a relaxation response that lessens cravings in opioid recovery patients.[36]

The National Acupuncture Detoxification Association (NADA), established in 1985, has developed an increasingly popular "acudetox" treatment strategy for addiction recovery. It offers, among other protocols, a three- to five-point auricular acupuncture protocol that has shown great effectiveness as an adjunct detoxification and relaxation therapy to help recovering addicts through withdrawal. Today more than 1,000 addiction treatment centers across the United States use the NADA protocol as an adjunctive therapy.[37]

The NADA acudetox protocol is not a stand-alone treatment; it is designed as an adjunct support treatment. However, the great benefit of the protocol is that it requires little training for practitioners compared to the 4 years of medical school that licensed acupuncturists are required to attend. This makes it an affordable and adaptable healing modality that can be easily implemented in opioid recovery centers.

After Withdrawal: Restoring Health

Acupuncture works by normalizing qi flow. If qi is stagnant, acupuncture gets it moving. If qi is imbalanced, acupuncture releases it from organs where it is excessive and brings it into organs where it is deficient. In this way, acupuncture restores balance and harmony to the organs, allowing our own self-healing mechanisms to work properly.

As we'll discuss throughout this book, opioids do a lot of damage to the body. The drugs themselves are toxic, causing physical injury to the brain, organs, and tissues. And the opioid habit causes poor health — users typically don't eat, sleep, or otherwise care for themselves very well. Thus, many people in recovery from opioid dependency face fatigue, nutritional deficits, neural deficits, organ damage, weak immune systems, and so on. Their health and vitality do not reappear immediately after withdrawal; recovery can be a long process.

Acupuncture can help with all of these issues. We'll discuss specific protocols in chapter 10. In particular, acupuncture is beneficial because it addresses health and vitality on both the physical and the emotional level. In Chinese medical theory (and increasingly in Western medical theory as well), the mind affects the body and the body affects the mind; the two are inseparable. Treating one while ignoring the other is a strategy for failure. Treating both, as acupuncture does, is the only path to true wellness.

COMPLEMENTARY THERAPIES

During an acupuncture session, a licensed acupuncturist may employ one or more of the following treatments:

Cupping

Cupping is a technique in which a glass cup is suctioned onto the body and allowed to sit for 10 to 20 minutes. This technique brings cellular waste to the surface of the skin, stimulating blood circulation and thus relieving swelling and pain. It is an ideal therapy for muscular pain.

Moxibustion

Moxibustion is the practice of burning mugwort (*Artemisia vulgaris*) above the skin. It is applied alone or with acupuncture to allow the heat to penetrate deeply into the acupoints. Moxibustion is typically applied in deficiency conditions. It can alleviate pain resulting from the stagnation of qi and blood created by cold conditions. It may also be used with those recovering from addiction who are experiencing prolonged fatigue.

Acupressure

Acupressure is the TCM practice of applying pressure, often using only the fingers, to key acupoints on the meridians to stimulate the body's natural self-curative abilities. It is a simple yet effective alternative to acupuncture that you can practice on yourself or another person. While the needling of acupuncture is generally thought to have a stronger effect than the simple application of pressure called for in acupressure, the advantage of acupressure is that it can be

Electrostimulation

In electrostimulation (E-stim), a small device produces an electrical current that passes through wires that are attached to the acupuncture needles by alligator clips. E-stim is typically used as an alternative to opioids in the management of pain caused by stagnations or deficiencies.

Tui Na

Tui na is a form of medical massage sometimes used to help increase the flow of blood and qi. It incorporates acupoints that can help balance or enhance the body's energies, and it can be used to manage pain and promote long-term wellness.

Medical Qi Gong

Emerging studies are showing the benefit of energy medicine in medical settings. Through the practice of healing touch, holistic practitioners manipulate patients' energetic fields to calm the nerves, release tension, and relieve pain.[38] Medical qi gong is similar to healing touch, but it is more intense and oriented around TCM theories; practitioners intentionally move qi and remove channel blocks to enhance patients' wellness.

done by the patient at home, several times per day, rather than requiring an office visit with a licensed acupuncturist. Multiple treatments per day culminate in a very powerful effect. You can combine acupressure with the application of essential oils to intensify the effect (see chapter 5).

Like any natural therapy, acupressure works quickly on acute conditions but will take regular long-term practice for chronic conditions.

Setting Intention

It is important to set your intention when performing acupressure. Avoid distractions. Applying acupressure while focusing your intent on the outcome will be much more effective than simply applying pressure to a point as you watch TV or talk on the phone.

Stimulating the Points

To energetically activate a healing point, apply pressure with your thumb or fingers. The pressure should be firm but not painful or uncomfortable. Massage the point for 1 to 3 minutes at a time.

Acupressure points are typically stimulated bilaterally (on each side of the body) unless they are located at the center of the body. Do not apply acupressure directly to areas of recent trauma; rather, treat the acupressure point on the opposite limb, or treat points above or below the affected area on the same channel.

Applying Essential Oils

To enhance the stimulation of a given acupoint, you can dilute and apply an appropriate essential oil to the point. (See chapter 5, where corresponding acupressure points are listed in the descriptions of essential oils indicated for recovery from opioid dependency.) You might, for example, apply an essential oil corresponding to the Water element (page 100) to a point on one of the channels corresponding to the Water element, such as the Kidney channel.

Acupressure and essential oils can be used separately or together during a treatment session.

Tonification versus Sedation

Acupressure can be performed for tonification or sedation. Tonification builds qi; sedation moves qi stagnation and reduces heat or toxins. When you apply pressure on an acupoint, use a slight clockwise motion on points for tonification; use a counterclockwise motion for sedating energy.

The two techniques can generally be applied to any point, but they would not both be used in the same session on the same point. You might, though, use each technique on different points in the same session. For example, suppose that you have recurring headaches. You are manifesting a pattern of Liver qi stagnation that causes Liver heat to rise to the head. At the same time, you have an underlying pattern of Kidney yin deficiency that is contributing to the Liver yin deficiency that is creating the stagnation and resulting heat there. In this situation, you would sedate acupoint LV 3 to relieve the stagnation and heat, and you would tonify acupoint KI 3 to restore yin. Together, the sedation and tonification will help resolve the headaches.

Acupoints for Opioid Dependency

Acupoints, as they're called, are located along the *channels* or *meridians* associated with the various organ systems. The channels are the riverways of qi in the body, and stimulating any point along them will facilitate the flow of qi and the function of the associated organ system. As we noted in chapter 2, each organ system is associated with a particular element; when you stimulate points on the channel of a particular organ system, you simultaneously stimulate that elemental influence in the body.

When trying to locate points for acupressure, know that they will often be more tender than the surrounding area, especially in fleshy parts of the body. Even trained acupuncturists will palpate an area to find a tender spot during treatments. Acupoints are typically in a dip rather than a bony protrusion.

In Chinese medicine, the body is measured by *cun* (pronounced "soon"), which is a unit that equals the width of the patient's thumb. The four fingers of the hand laid flat equal three cun.

Following are some of the most effective points for opioid dependency: they reduce cravings, alleviate withdrawal symptoms, and ease pain. I have chosen them because of their effectiveness and because they are easy for a novice to locate.

For help in locating these acupoints, turn to the illustrations beginning on page 62.

Acupoints for the Water Element

Essential oils corresponding with the Water element (page 100) can be diluted and applied to activate points on the Kidney (KI) and Bladder (BL) meridians, with or without pressure.

KI 3 *Location:* On the inside of the ankle, on the medial aspect (middle) of the foot, in the depression between the end of the medial malleolus (the prominence on the inside of the ankle formed by the base of the tibia) and the ankle tendon.

Tonification: KI 3 is the source point for the Kidney organ system and is an important point for any yin or yang deficiencies. It especially nourishes yin and clears heat resulting from yin deficiency. It fortifies the immune system and the metabolism. Used for adrenal fatigue in addiction recovery and for sweats experienced during withdrawal. Also used for chronic pain of the knee or lower back and for acute ankle and heel pain.

KI 6 *Location:* On the inside of the ankle, on the medial aspect of the foot, in the dip below the end of the medial malleolus.

Tonification: KI 6 is one of the best points to nourish Kidney yin and is used together with LU 7 for breathing issues such as asthma, the inability to catch your breath, dry throat, and dry cough. It helps calm shen in cases of emotional disorders.

BL 2 *Location:* On the face, on the inner border of the eyebrow in the depression on the medial end of the supraorbital notch (the small groove in the bony path that runs along the eye socket).

Sedation: Indicated for watering or twitching eyes during withdrawal or hiccups. Calms headache along the forehead, eyebrows, or eyes. A minor point for mania.

BL 60 *Location:* On the foot behind the outside of the ankle in the depression between the tip of the lateral malleolus (the prominence on the outside of the ankle formed by the base of the fibula) and the tendon.

Tonification: Used in cases of acute lower back pain, stiff neck, and sciatica with pain that radiates down the middle of the posterior (back) side of the leg or calf. Also used for leg spasms experienced during withdrawal.

Sedation: Used to address acute dizziness, headaches, eye pain, or mania.

BL 62 *Location:* On the outside of the ankle in the depression directly below the lateral malleolus.

Tonification: Calms the shen when there are emotional upsets or insomnia. Eases pain of the lower back and back of the leg. Used with SI 3 for headaches, upper back and neck pain, or tinnitus (ringing of the ears).

Acupoints for the Wood Element

Essential oils corresponding with the Wood element (page 100) can be diluted and applied to activate acupoints on the Liver (LV) and Gallbladder (GB) meridians, with or without pressure.

LV 2 *Location:* On the top of the foot between the tendons of the big toe and second toe.

Sedation: Strongly clears Liver heat attributed to prolonged Liver qi stagnation with indications such as insomnia with vivid dreams; red, swollen, and painful eyes; and aggressive outbursts of anger. Also helpful for acute headaches brought on by stress and frustration.

LV 3 *Location:* On the dorsum (upper surface) of the foot, in the depression proximal (next) to the first metatarsal space.

Tonification: Used to nourish Liver blood and Liver yin. Also used with LI 4 for pain anywhere in the body, as the coupling of these four acupressure points (called the Four Gates) moves qi and blood throughout the body.

Sedation: Indicated for headaches; dizziness; redness, swelling, or pain of the face; a feeling of abdominal or rib area distention; hiccups or digestive upset due to Liver overacting on the Spleen. Also can help ease emotional upset, anger, stress, aggression, and sleep disturbances.

GB 1
Location: On the face just on the side of the eye, at the outer canthus of the lateral side of the eye socket (the angle formed at the meeting of the upper and lower eyelids).

Sedation: Used for watering eyes during withdrawal and for headaches, especially at the temples.

GB 20
Location: At the base of the skull on the nape, below the occiput (the back part of the skull) in a depression between the upper portion of the sternocleidomastoideus and trapezius muscles (two large neck muscles).

Sedation: Indicated for headaches, eye pain, neck pain. Helps to lower blood pressure.

GB 34
Location: On the leg, below the knee, on the lateral (outer) aspect in the depression anterior and inferior to (behind and below) the head of the fibula.

Tonification: Used for leg spasms experienced during withdrawal and for pain in the joint or arthritis. For pain along the GB channel, or pain running down the lateral side of the leg, and sciatica radiating down the outside of the leg; swelling and/or pain of the knee or lower leg or foot; and pain due to sprains anywhere in the body. Also used for pain related to gallbladder disease.

GB 40
Location: On the foot below the ankle, anterior and inferior to the external malleolus.

Tonification: Indicated for weakness in the lower legs or foot; for pain along the GB channel, or pain running down the lateral side of the leg and sciatica radiating down the outside of the leg; and for ankle pain or swelling. For ankle sprains or injury, treat the opposite ankle rather than the injured ankle.

Sedation: Indicated for Liver qi stagnation; helps to soothe the Liver and pain or distention over or below the ribs.

GB 41 *Location:* On the top of the foot, lateral and proximal to the fourth metatarsophalangeal joint (between the foot and the toe), in the depression distal to the junction of the 4th and 5th metatarsal bones, on the lateral side of m. extensor digitorum longus.

Sedation: Pulls down excessive Liver yang energies resulting in headaches, red eyes, tearing eyes, and migraines. Breaks up Liver congestion and alleviates anger and frustration. Eases pain or spasms of the fourth and fifth toes or top of the foot. For acute injuries in the area of GB 41, treat the opposite foot rather than the injured foot. Treats any pain of the chest. Combine with TB 5 for temporal or one-sided headaches.

Acupoints for the Fire Element

Essential oils corresponding with the Fire element (page 100) can be diluted and applied to activate acupoints on the Heart (HT), Pericardium (PER), Triple Burner (TB) and Small Intestine (SI) meridians, with or without pressure.

HT 5 *Location:* On the inside of the wrist, on the radial side of the flexor carpi ulnaris muscle, 1 cun above the crease of the wrist (dividing the arm from the hand).

Tonification: Helps to normalize heart rhythm and can pacify severe palpitations. Subdues chronic yawning experienced during withdrawal. Can help with sudden loss of voice or tongue stiffness. Indicated for pain of the wrist, elbow, and fourth and fifth fingers. Calms the shen.

HT 6 *Location:* On the inside of the wrist, on the radial side of the tendon of the flexor carpi ulnaris muscle, 0.5 cun above the crease of the wrist.

Tonification: Used for fever and night sweats during acute opioid withdrawal, as well as for deep sensations of bone pain. Also used for cardiac pain and palpitations associated with panic and fright during withdrawal.

HT 7 *Location:* On the inside of the wrist, on radial side of the tendon of the flexor carpi ulnaris muscle, on the crease of the wrist.

Tonification: Calms the shen to ease emotional upset, insomnia, and frightful dreams. HT 7 is the source point for the Heart and reinforces all Heart-related functions while calming palpitation. This is an excellent point for recovering addicts who find themselves lashing out at others.

HT 8 *Location:* On the palm, on the crease between the fourth and fifth metacarpal bones, where the tip of the little finger touches when a fist is made.

Sedation: Indicated for severe insomnia or, for those who are able to sleep, for nightmares. Calms shen disturbances due to Heart fire.

SI 3 *Location:* When a loose fist is made, the point is on the outside of the hand just below the knuckle of the pinky finger where the red and white skin intersect, on the ulnar aspect proximal to the fifth metacarpophalangeal joint (between the hand and the finger).

Tonification: Indicated for pain and rigidity of the head and neck, especially when there is pain turning the head from side to side. Eases pain anywhere along the SI channel, including the scapula area. Combine with BL 62 for tremors and spasms in the arms and legs associated with detoxing or recovery, alternating chills/sweats, and watering eyes. Combine with BL 62 for leg, knee, spine, or low back pain.

PER 6 *Location:* On the palm side of the forearm, 2 cun above the crease of the wrist between the tendons of the palmaris longus muscle and the flexor carpi radialis muscle.

Tonification: Calms the mind and is useful with insomnia and those who are easily startled. Regulates heart rhythm and eases palpitations. Opens the chest and is used for coughs, breathing difficulties, and asthma. Eases symptoms of depression and enhances cognition. Used for pain associated with bending the elbow. This is the famous point used for seasickness. It is very effective for nausea, hiccups, and vomiting associated with detox and recovery, especially when combined with SP 4.

PER 7

Location: On the palm side of the crease of the wrist between the tendons of the palmaris longus muscle and the flexor carpi radialis muscle.

Tonification: Used in detoxification during withdrawal; eases sweating, sighing, stomach pain, nausea/vomiting, insomnia, and emotional upset. Also helpful for pain of the elbows, wrist pain, and splitting headaches. Used to treat the crying-and-laughing fits seen during withdrawal as well as shortness of breath.

PER 8

Location: In the center of the palm, between the second and third metacarpal bones, where the tip of the middle finger touches when a fist is made.

Sedation: Used to clear Heart fire with symptoms seen in opioid cessation such as mania, mouth and tongue ulcers, cardiac pain (call 911 with a cardiac event), violent emotional outbursts, inability to sleep through the night, and night terrors. Eases the ceaseless restlessness seen during withdrawal, as well as hand tremors and sweating palms.

TB 5

Location: On the back of the forearm on the dorsal aspect 2 cun above the transverse crease of the wrist between the ulna and the radius.

Tonification: Indicated for pain along the TB channel, as well as pain of the elbow, neck, and upper back. Eases pain and ringing in the ears, swelling and pain of the cheek and teeth, and pain and swelling of the hand, wrist, and fingers. Combined with GB 41, it is used to alleviate pain in any joint, tightness and pain at the area joining the shoulders and neck, and pain along the ribs. Used for dizziness, headaches, or eye pain with a sudden onset.

Acupoints for the Earth Element

Essential oils corresponding with the Earth element (page 100) can be diluted and applied to activate acupoints on the Spleen (SP) and Stomach (ST) meridians, with or without pressure.

SP 3

Location: Beside and below the big-toe joint on the inside of the foot at the junction of the red and white skin, on the medial side in the depression posterior and inferior to the proximal metatarsodigital joint.

Tonification: Used for any condition related to Spleen qi deficiency, including digestive issues, gastric or epigastric pain, abdominal distension, and diarrhea. Indicated in early stages of recovery from addiction when there are hunger pangs but no true desire to eat. Used for boosting qi in cases of fatigue or weakness following detox.

SP 4

Location: On the inside arch of the foot, in the depression distal and inferior to (outside and beneath) the base of the first metatarsal bone.

Tonification: Indicated for acute stomach pain, abdominal/ rib distention and fullness, poor appetite, vomiting, and diarrhea. Combine with PER 6 for insomnia, restlessness, and emotional upset. For women, the two-point combination also alleviates PMS and menstrual pain following opioid dependence.

SP 6

Location: On the inside of the lower leg, 3 cun above the medial malleolus, on the posterior (back) border of the medial aspect of the tibia.

Tonification: Indicated for acute stomach pain, abdominal heaviness, no desire to eat, vomiting of clear fluids, and diarrhea with undigested food. Treats pain anywhere along the Spleen channel. For men, used along with LV 2 to subdue sexual hyperactivity, pain in the penis, and nocturnal sperm emissions following prolonged drug use that has resulted in chronic Liver heat.

SP 9 *Location:* Below the knee on the medial aspect of the lower leg, in the depression of the lower border of the medial condyle of the tibia (the projection at the top of that bone).

Tonification: Treats dampness (see Spleen qi deficiency, page 160) with indications such as pain that worsens in damp weather, a heavy feeling in the body, poor cognition with a foggy brain, and the inability to wake in the morning.

ST 36 *Location:* On outside of the lower leg, on the anterior aspect (front), 3 cun below the kneecap and 1 cun from the anterior crest of the tibia.

Tonification: Arguably one of the most popular and useful acupoints. Used for any pain or problems associated with the stomach, digestion or indigestion, constipation, or poor appetite. Calms the mind and shen, and is used with all types of emotional disorders. Boosts qi energy, nourishes blood and yin, and restores vitality. Normalizes and boosts the immune system and generally promotes wellness. Treats pain anywhere along the Stomach channel.

ST 44 *Location:* On the top of the foot, proximal to the web margin between the second and third toes, at the junction of the red and white skin.

Sedation: Clears heat from the ST channel with symptoms such as toothache, pain of the face or eyes, and nosebleed.

Acupoints for the Metal Element

Essential oils corresponding with the Metal element (page 100) can be diluted and applied to activate acupoints on the Lungs (LU) and Large Intestine (LI) meridians, with or without pressure.

LU 5 *Location:* On the cubital crease (the inside of the elbow), on the radial side of the tendon of the biceps brachii muscle.

Tonification: Used for pain along the Lung channel, upper arm, and elbow. Eases spasmodic pain of the elbow and arm, difficulty opening the hand, and shoulder pain with difficulty raising the hand to the head. Also used for acute intestinal spasms and pain, as well as abdominal pain with vomiting and diarrhea. Treats alternating fever and sweats, sneezing, shivering, and uncontrollable crying during withdrawal. Strongly indicated for coughing, wheezing, and shortness of breath.

LU 7

Location: On the forearm 1.5 cun above the wrist crease on the radial margin of the forearm, superior to (above) the styloid process of the radius (the projection of bone at the wrist).

Tonification: Indicated for head and neck pain, including migraines (central and one-sided), headaches, and neck rigidity. Also used for toothache, cough, asthma, and pain in the genitals.

LU 9

Location: On the crease of the wrist, below the thumb where the radial artery pulsates.

Tonification: Reinforces the Lungs due to any imbalance or deficiency, including coughing with a large amount of phlegm and asthma with wheezing. Used in detoxification for acute feelings of chest compression and shortness of breath as well as hiccups that will not cease. Used for pain of the wrist and thumb.

LI 4

Location: On the top of the hand between the thumb and the pointer finger, between the first and second metacarpal bones, in the middle of the second metacarpal bone on the radial side.

Tonification: When combined with LV 3 (together they are called the Four Gates), can be used to treat pain anywhere in the body by moving qi and blood. Treats pain of the head and face, headaches, swelling and pain of the eye, and toothache in the lower jaw. Regulates immune response and restores warmth to the body.

LI 11 *Location:* On the lateral (outside) end of the transverse cubital crease (the crease of the elbow), found with the elbow flexed.

Sedation: Used to treat feelings of heat in the body, fever, and the hot skin/itching sometimes experienced with opioid withdrawal. Treats pain, numbness, weakness, and swelling. Eases spasms and contractions of the elbow, shoulder, arm, and hand; also used for spasms along the entire Large Intestine channel.

Supplementary Points

The Conception Vessel (CV) is an acupuncture channel that traverses the middle of the anterior trunk. It is not associated with the five elements but impacts many diverse functions of the body. CV points are easy for a novice to find, making them helpful in self-treatment.

CV 6 *Location:* 1.5 cun below the belly button.
Tonification: Used for tonifying the qi and yang of the whole body. Helpful for recovering strength and vitality following opioid dependence.

CV 12 *Location:* On the stomach, on the middle line of the upper abdomen, 4 cun above the belly button.
Tonification: Used for quelling stomach upset, epigastric pain, vomiting, hiccups, and acid regurgitation.

Acupoints Illustrated

WATER ELEMENT MERIDIANS

KIDNEY (KI)

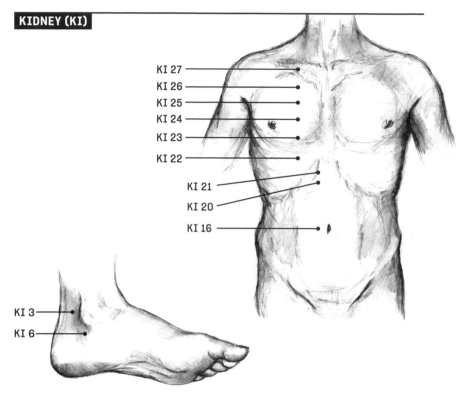

KI 27
KI 26
KI 25
KI 24
KI 23
KI 22
KI 21
KI 20
KI 16

KI 3
KI 6

BLADDER (BL)

BL 2

BL 60
BL 62

WOOD ELEMENT MERIDIANS

LIVER (LV)

GALLBLADDER (GB)

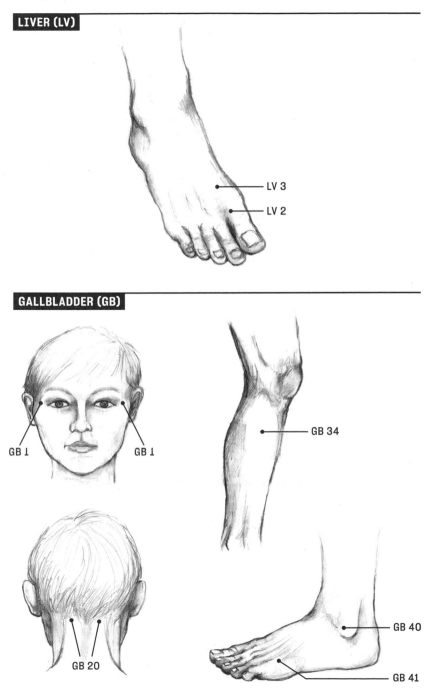

Acupoints Illustrated *continued*

FIRE ELEMENT MERIDIANS

HEART (HT)

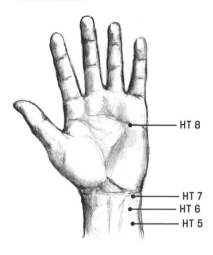

HT 8

HT 7
HT 6
HT 5

SMALL INTESTINE (SI)

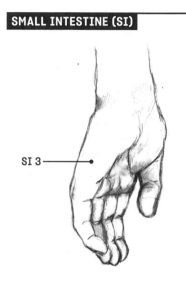

SI 3

PERICARDIUM (PER)

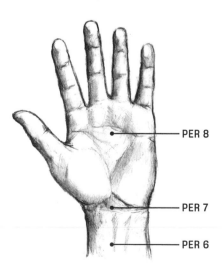

PER 8

PER 7

PER 6

TRIPLE BURNER (TB)

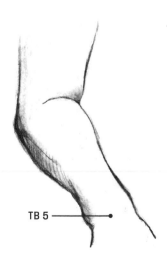

TB 5

EARTH ELEMENT MERIDIANS

SPLEEN (SP)

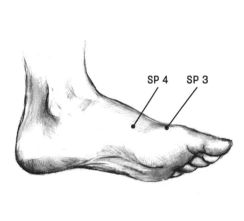

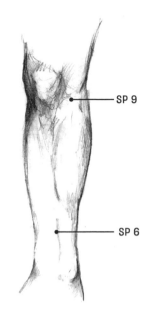

SP 4   SP 3

SP 9

SP 6

STOMACH (ST)

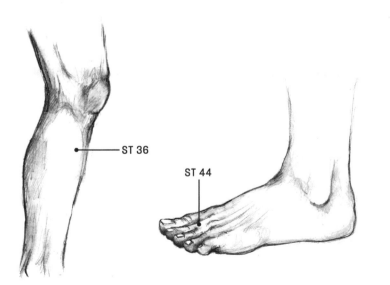

ST 36

ST 44

Acupoints Illustrated *continued*
METAL ELEMENT MERIDIANS

LUNGS (LU)

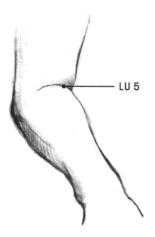

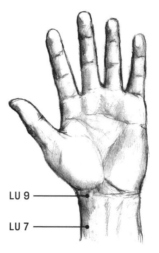

LU 5

LU 9

LU 7

LARGE INTESTINE (LI)

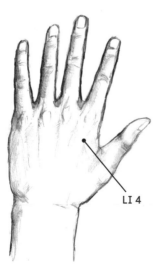

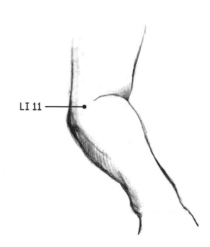

LI 11

LI 4

SUPPLEMENTARY

CONCEPTION VESSEL (CV)

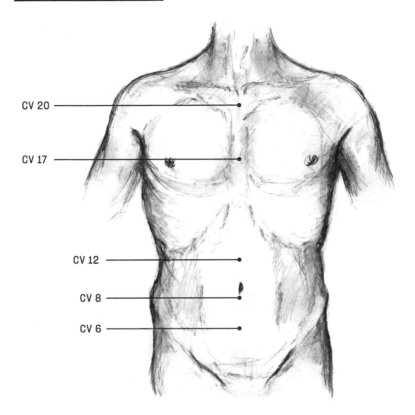

CV 20

CV 17

CV 12

CV 8

CV 6

CHAPTER 4

Herbs
Powerful Plant Medicines
to Drive Recovery

Herbs offer powerful medicine for anyone recovering from opioid
dependency. From herbs that help the body manage pain and
support heart healing to those that tonify the body and invigorate
the immune system, these botanical medicines can play a vital role in
helping opioid users through the withdrawal and recovery processes.

Traditional Chinese medicine generally calls for complex herb
formulas that synthesize the healing effects of many plants. These formulas provide a much stronger action than single herbs by themselves.
However, Chinese herbs are hard to obtain in the United States, and
learning to use them in formulas requires training. If you decide to use
the Chinese herb formulas cited in this book, I recommend that you
consult with a trained TCM practitioner; he or she will have access to
the herbs and can prepare the formulas for you.

Thankfully, many widely available herbs that are used in Western
herbal medicine have potent applications for treating opioid dependency. We'll talk about these herbs and their uses in this chapter. You
can use them as needed, or you can incorporate them as elements in a

larger treatment protocol (see part 2 of this book for examples). For guidance on which herbs might work best for your specific situation, consult with a trained Western herbalist.

Herbs for Targeting Opioid Dependency

For the purposes of this book, I have chosen to highlight the following categories of herbs that are particularly useful in facilitating recovery from opioid dependency:

CATEGORY OF ACTION	EXAMPLES	
TONIC HERBS	astragalus	goji
	atractylodes	jiao gu lan
	codonopsis	reishi
	fo-ti	
NERVINES	California poppy	passionflower
	lemon balm	skullcap
	lavender	wild lettuce
ADAPTOGENS	ashwagandha	
	codonopsis	
	eleuthero	
	jiao gu lan	
DETOXIFICATION HERBS	burdock	
	dandelion	
	yellow dock	
IMMUNE SUPPORT HERBS	astragalus	eleuthero
	atractylodes	jiao gu lan
	burdock	privet fruit
	codonopsis	reishi
	elecampane	

CATEGORY OF ACTION	EXAMPLES	
PAIN RELIEF HERBS	atractylodes	passionflower
	California poppy	red sage
	cannabis	turmeric
	elecampane	white peony
	kratom	wild lettuce
	meadowsweet	willow
	motherwort	yarrow
	mullein	
HEART HEALTH HERBS	elecampane	hawthorn
	fo-ti	motherwort
	goji	red sage
LUNG HEALTH HERBS	codonopsis	
	elecampane	
	goji	
	mullein	
LIVER HEALTH HERBS	burdock	red sage
	dandelion	schisandra
	fo-ti	turmeric
	goji	white peony
	jiao gu lan	yellow dock
	privet fruit	
PSYCHOACTIVE HERBS	cannabis	
	kratom	

Let's take a quick look at what these different categories of action encompass, followed by a look at the different kinds of preparations used in herbal medicine, and then I'll offer brief profiles of the herbs listed above, specifically focusing on their applications for opioid dependency.

Tonic Herbs

Tonic herbs are more of a superfood than a medicine. They support the health of an entire organ system or the entire body by supporting balance and harmony of energies. They work over the long term and must be taken for an extended period to have an effect.

Most of the medicinal herbs you will run into at your local health food store are designed to address certain diseases or imbalances and are intended for short-term use. You might, for example, take echinacea for a week to help fight off a cold. In contrast, you might consume a tonic herb such as codonopsis year-round to strengthen your immune system so that you are not susceptible to a cold in the first place.

Tonic herbs share several characteristics that make them appropriate for people who are recovering from opioid dependency. In particular, they have the following uses:

- Supplementing deficient yin or yang in the body

- Providing the nutrients necessary to restore or nourish specific organ systems

- Supporting the blood and shen, qi, and jing

- Strengthening the immune system

Nervines

Nervine herbs impart an immediate calming effect, which can be helpful for anyone experiencing the anxiety, jitteriness, tension, cravings, and other physical and emotional symptoms of stress as they go through withdrawal from opioids. Though they are not as strong as pharmaceutical opioids, they do take the edge off.

Adaptogens

Adaptogenic herbs are amazing for opioid dependency. They help us adapt to stress, and the one thing that overcoming an opioid dependency invariably creates is stress. We must reconsider family dynamics, career choices, and survival modalities during the recovery period.

Adaptogenic herbs help smooth out all of our physical and emotional responses during this tumultuous time.

Detoxification Herbs

Opioids are themselves toxic substances, and they place a burden on the organs of detoxification. Many people who are looking to free themselves from opioid dependency find that detoxification herbs, which encourage the release of toxins from the body, can help them bring their body back into balance and prepare to heal. Use detox herbs with care, as they are cold in nature and clear heat from the body. Though clearing heat is useful for detoxifying, the cold influence can exacerbate a yin-yang imbalance or damage Spleen qi if it is excessive.

Immune Support Herbs

Long-term opioid abuse has been linked to a reduced immune response.[39] According to Chinese medicine, the simple fact that people who abuse opioids do not eat well, sleep well, or generally care for themselves would result in a lowered immune response. The herbs profiled here support and strengthen the immune system to help people in recovery regain their innate defenses against illness.

Pain Relief Herbs

Though herbs are not as powerful as opioids in relieving pain, they remain an effective natural strategy for pain reduction without any significant risk or side effects. Some herbs are taken internally for their therapeutic benefits, and some can be used topically as analgesics. See page 185 for more details.

Heart Health Herbs

The herbs profiled here nourish and strengthen the Heart, qi and boost the circulation of blood. Heart health is often damaged by opioid abuse, and these herbs can play an important role in reversing that damage. See page 156 for more details.

Lung Health Herbs

Because opioid abuse often translates to qi deficiency, which contributes to internal dampness, and to immune deficiency, which leaves the body vulnerable to pathogens, the lungs are vulnerable to damp accumulations and infections in opioid users. In addition, cigarette smoking is prevalent among people recovering from opioid addiction, which obviously is another debilitating factor for the lungs.[40] For these reasons, herbs that support and repair the lungs can be an important part of a recovery program.

Liver Health Herbs

Liver damage has not been directly linked to prescription doses of opioids. However, overdose of opioids can cause acute liver injury, and opioids are often taken in combination with acetaminophen, which does damage the liver. The U.S. National Institutes of Health explains, "A special form of liver injury linked to opioid use occurs with their fixed drug combinations with acetaminophen. These combinations are commonly used for moderate to moderately severe pain and can lead to abuse. If taken too frequently, acetaminophen doses may reach toxic levels."[41] The herbs profiled here can be used to purge the liver of toxins, to repair liver tissue, and to restore the proper function of the liver.

Psychoactive Herbs

More than 63,600 people died of drug overdoses in 2016, up 21 percent from year before, according to data released by the U.S. National Center for Health Statistics. This is partly due to the fact that deaths from synthetic, nonmethadone opioids like fentanyl (which is 50 to 100 times stronger than heroin) climbed steeply in 2016.[42] Psychoactive herbs can play an important role in helping people overcome opioid dependency by serving as alternative, less risky stimulants that users are more easily able to give up over time. While these herbs do carry the potential to become habitual substances themselves, the risks associated with their use pale in comparison to those of opioid use. In our battle against serious opioid addiction, I feel that these herbs must be considered.

REALISTIC EXPECTATIONS

I have read several posts online by people who are trying to give up an opioid dependency and are disappointed that an herb formula they are trying does not replace their opioid medication. This is not how herbs are meant to be used. First, you cannot expect herbs to replace narcotics wholesale; herbs are meant to be used as part of a larger holistic treatment plan. Nervine-type herbs can be calming, but the effect is going to be gentler than that of opioids. Adaptogens can be used to rewire the brain and heal neurological damage, but they will take weeks or months to work. Tonic herbs and those that support the immune system and organ systems also take many months to work. While herbs can be a vital part of a full recovery and restore true emotional and physical wellness, realistic expectations must prevail.

Herbal Remedies: A Breakdown of the Different Preparations

Herbs are available in many different forms, and the dosage instructions will vary depending on the form you're using. This book focuses on dried herbs, which is what you'll most often find commercially. We'll talk here about the different forms of prepared herbal medicines you can buy, but of course you can also buy dried herbs in bulk and make your own medicines. There are many good reference books available to show you how.

Unless otherwise stated, the dosages noted in the profiles in this chapter assume that you will be using dried plant material and preparing the dosages for average-size adults.

TCM Clinic Formulas

Clinic formulas are concentrated powdered extracts of many herbs mixed together in a precise ratio. They are typically found in a 1:5 concentration — that is, five parts of the original plant material went into making one part of the powder. They are called "clinic formulas" because they are prepared according to a formula given by a clinic practitioner — in North America, this is generally a licensed acupuncturist. I give my own clinic formulas in the protocols in part 2 of this book. Follow your acupuncturist's instructions for dosages.

Advantages: The ratios can be modified for individual patients. The powders can be added to liquids or smoothies for those who have trouble swallowing pills.

Disadvantages: You will taste the herbs. The concentrated powders are rarely available in organic form.

TCM Patent Formulas

Patent formulas are the classic herb formulas that all students of TCM learn. These are time-tested remedies that have been used for generations. You can often buy them from herb shops and online suppliers.

Advantages: Patent remedies are often inexpensive and are convenient to use.

Disadvantages: Patent remedies are most commonly made in China, and there is growing concern about heavy metals, adulterants, and pesticides found in these products.[43] Try to source patent remedies made from certified organic ingredients produced in the United States.

Capsules

Capsules are usually obtained from commercial sources, though you can make your own if you have empty capsules and finely powdered herbs. As for commercial capsules, dosages vary, because some capsules contain simply powdered dried herbs, whereas others contain concentrated powdered herbs.

Advantages: Capsules are easy to find. In swallowing them, you do not have to taste bitter herbs.

Disadvantages: Capsules are of varying quality, and therapeutic doses are costly. Some capsules contain fillers, making them less potent for the high cost.

Tablets

Like capsules, tablets often can be purchased from commercial sources. However, you can make them at home as well: Combine 1 cup of powdered herbs and ¼ cup of brown rice flour. Add enough water to give the mixture the consistency of pie crust dough. Pinch off small bits, roll them into tiny balls, place them on a cookie sheet, and bake at 175°F (90°C) for 2 hours. Put the tablets in a cool, dark place to dry; when they are completely dry, store them in a glass jar in a cool, dark spot.

Advantages: Tablets are convenient to use. When swallowing them, you do not have to taste bitter herbs.

Disadvantages: Homemade tablets are time-consuming to prepare, and dosage can be unpredictable. Commercial tablets may have undesirable ingredients used as binders, fillers, or coatings.

Infusions and Decoctions

Infusions and decoctions are medicinal-strength teas. You can purchase premixed formulas at herb shops and natural food stores, or you can make your own. Typically you'll use anywhere from ½ to 1 ounce of dried herbs per 4 cups of water. An infusion is made from leaves, flowers, and other delicate parts of a plant that need only be steeped in hot water to extract their constituents. A decoction is made from roots, bark, seeds, and other tough plant parts that need to be boiled to extract their constituents. Once you've made the tea, add honey, if desired, and sip it throughout the day. It will keep for up to 3 days in the refrigerator.

To make an infusion, bring water to a boil, then pour it over your dried herbs. Cover and let steep for approximately 20 minutes. Strain the tea and drink it warm or cold; add honey if desired.

To make a decoction, combine the dried herbs and water in a saucepan and bring to a boil. Cover and let simmer for 20 minutes, then strain the tea and drink.

Advantages: Infusions and decoctions typically cost less than prepared remedies. You can control the quality of plant material and sometimes find organic herbs domestically. Making tea is very ritualistic; this can help replace some of the ritualistic activities associated with drug use.

Disadvantages: The taste of herbs can sometimes be unpleasant.

Tinctures

Tinctures are alcoholic extracts of herbs. You can buy them at health food stores, herb shops, and online. You can also make your own: Finely chop or powder dried herbs and put them in a glass jar. Add enough 80-proof vodka to cover the herbs. Typically you'd use a 1:5 ratio of dried herbs to vodka; that is, for every 1 ounce of dried herbs, you'd use 5 ounces of vodka. Cover the jar and let steep in a cool, dark spot for 2 weeks. Shake daily. Then strain out the herbs.

A tincture is very potent medicine. The standard dose for a 160-pound adult is usually 2 ml three to five times daily. This can vary greatly depending on the strength of the herb and the duration of use. You can dilute a dose of tincture in water or juice for palatability.

Advantages: Tinctures retain their potency for many years and are a convenient method for extracting and storing a plant's medicinal constituents.

Disadvantages: Many people who are recovering from opioid addiction may also have issues with alcohol. This would not be an ideal type of remedy for those whose cravings are triggered by alcohol.

Glycerites

A glycerite is made like a tincture, except the herbal extract is made with diluted vegetable glycerin instead of alcohol. With dried herbs, you'd use a ratio of about 1 part herbs to 5 parts liquid, and that liquid would be 60 percent glycerin and 40 percent purified water. With fresh herbs, you'd use a 1:1 ratio of herbs to liquid, and the liquid would be about 90 percent glycerin and 10 percent purified water. Glycerites have a higher risk of developing mold than alcohol tinctures do, so make sure that the herbs are completely covered by the diluted glycerin.

An adult dosage would be around 2 teaspoons three to five times daily. Glycerites are very sweet and can be taken directly under the tongue. Although this is a stable mixture, it should be stored for only 6 to 12 months.

Advantages: Glycerites have a sweet flavor and are easy to administer or consume

Disadvantages: They are costly to purchase and time-consuming to make.

MAKING HERBAL MEDICINES AT HOME

Here are a few points to always remember when making herbal medicines:

- Avoid aluminum, plastic, or iron equipment and utensils when making herbal medicines. Glass, wood, stainless steel, and enamel are better choices.

- Always label and date your medicine and note where the herb came from.

- Keep your homemade remedies away from heat and direct sunlight.

Medicinal Herbs: Profiles

The herbs profiled here are those that I consider to be most useful
for combating opioid dependency, whether during withdrawal
or recovery. Many have a wide range of actions and offer aid on
multiple fronts. Again, unless otherwise noted, the dosages given
in these profiles are for average-size adults and assume that you are
taking dried plant material.

Ashwagandha

BOTANICAL NAME: *Withania somnifera*

PART USED: root

DOSE: 2–4 grams daily

Ashwagandha has been studied extensively for its ability to reduce
anxiety and stress. A review of five human trials concluded that it
is an effective adaptogen.[44] It has been proved a reliable remedy for
stress, debility, nervous exhaustion, insomnia, and loss of memory.
It has also been proved to enhance cognitive function; apparently,
it enhances the function of brain's receptor sites.[45] It has even been
shown to help control weight for stressed individuals struggling
with obesity.[46]

The root can be brewed as a standard decoction, but in the
Ayurvedic tradition it is traditionally prepared as a milk decoction
with honey to promote a deep sleep and to revive those with chronic
debility or dullness of the mind. You can also take it in the form of
capsules, tablets, or tinctures.

Astragalus (Huang Qi)

BOTANICAL NAME: *Astragalus membranaceus*

PART USED: root

DOSE: 1–3 grams daily

Astragalus has long been used to treat immune system disorders, inflammatory diseases, and cancer.[47] It is a specific qi tonic for wound healing, making it especially helpful for people with wounds and sores that are slow to heal, a factor often seen with recovering addicts. While astragalus is not a stimulant, like caffeine, it does help increase energy. Some people find that taking it late in the day interferes with sleep, so take it before 2:00 p.m.

Astragalus root is commonly consumed in the form of capsules, tablets, decoctions, or tinctures. Try simmering a few slices of the root in broth and sipping it throughout the morning.

Atractylodes (Bai Zhu)

BOTANICAL NAME: *Atractylodes macrocephala*

PART USED: root

DOSE: 2–4 grams daily

Atractylodes is a highly revered Spleen qi tonic used for all types of Spleen qi deficiency and internal dampness. Atractylodes is gaining much attention for its ability to modulate blood sugar and improve the body's ability to use insulin on a cellular level;[48] it would be appropriate to use at any stage of diabetes.

Atractylodes is also known to be an immune system modulator, and it is seeing use in the treatment of cancer.[49] Recent studies have identified neuroprotective properties in the herb that may help preserve and enhance cognition.[50] It is traditionally included in pain formulas both taken internally and applied topically; it is believed to have anti-inflammatory qualities.[51]

Atractylodes is commonly taken in the form of capsules, tablets, decoctions, or tinctures.

Burdock (Gobo)

BOTANICAL NAME: *Arctium lappa*

PART USED: root

DOSE: 4–8 grams daily

Burdock root has long been used as a blood cleanser and cancer remedy in Western herbalism. Scientific studies of burdock have been able to isolate in it the chemical compound arctigenin, which starves cancer cells of glucose.[52] One study has suggested that, due to its antioxidant qualities, burdock root can protect the liver from damage due to alcohol abuse; since opioids, too, are processed by the liver, one might surmise that it can be of assistance in cases of opioid abuse as well.[53] Similarly, it has been suggested that burdock root can assist in the treatment of diabetes, and because opioid abuse results in metabolic damage and blood-sugar issues, burdock remains an interesting remedy for those in opioid recovery.[54]

Burdock root can be cooked and eaten like carrots; it's a common addition to medicinal soups. You can also take it in the form of capsules, tablets, decoctions, or tinctures.

California Poppy

BOTANICAL NAME: *Eschscholzia californica*

PART USED: dry aerial parts

DOSE: 2–3 grams daily

This is a valuable plant in helping opioid users through the withdrawal process. It can be used to help induce sleep, reduce pain, and calm the mind. Though it is related to the opium poppy from which opioid drugs like heroin are made, the California poppy contains different forms of alkaloids with milder sedative and pain-relieving qualities.

California poppy is easily prepared as an infusion, and it is also commonly taken in the form of capsules, tablets, and tinctures.

Cannabis

BOTANICAL NAME: *Cannabis sativa*

PARTS USED: leaves, flower buds

DOSE: varies depending on the strain

Cannabis offers a viable alternative to opioids in the treatment of pain. In a comprehensive 2017 report, the Health and Medicine Division of the National Academies of Sciences, Engineering, and Medicine stated, "There is conclusive or substantial evidence that cannabis or cannabinoids are effective . . . for the treatment of chronic pain in adults."[55] A study published in that same year stated, "Introducing cannabis into the treatment of chronic pain may result in a reduction or complete cessation of opioid use thereby significantly reducing the potential for dependence or overdose."[56] Another study noted a 64 percent decrease in opioid use among medical marijuana patients and a 45 percent improvement in quality of life.[57]

Cannabis is typically smoked or consumed as an edible. Smoking carries the risk of carcinogens, so edibles are preferred.

Caution: Cannabis use is not without its risks, though they are minor compared to the potential risks associated with opioids.[58] According to TCM, prolonged cannabis use dulls the shen (spirit). This is evident with a lack of motivation, the inability to perform strategic life planning, and the inability to see plans through to fruition. This leads to a life of unfulfilled potential. While this scenario is not optimal, opioid addiction has greater risks, such as brain damage and overdose. Comparably, cannabis is the far lesser evil of the two and should be considered a viable option in possible strategies to combat the opioid crisis.

Codonopsis (Dang Shen)

BOTANICAL NAME: *Codonopsis pilosula*

PART USED: root

DOSE: 4–8 grams daily

Ginseng is a well-known qi tonic, but it can be overstimulating for someone battling an opioid dependency. Codonopsis root closely mimics ginseng's tonic qualities while expressing a gentler, nourishing effect. It replenishes qi while also supporting the Spleen and promoting Lung function. Codonopsis is also an exceptional blood tonic and a key immune system tonic, as it helps to build both red blood cell counts and white blood cell counts.[59] It also acts as an adaptogen, increasing the body's ability to adapt to stressors. Promising research has shown that its immune-stimulating and anti-inflammatory properties may help the body combat both cancer and chronic obstructive pulmonary disease (COPD).[60]

Codonopsis is commonly taken in the form of capsules, tablets, decoctions, or tinctures. You can also use it in medicinal soups; strain it out before consuming the soup.

Dandelion

BOTANICAL NAME: *Taraxacum officinale*

PART USED: root

DOSE: 1–3 grams daily

Dandelion root is used in TCM for all types of Liver disorders, such as cirrhosis and hepatitis involving heat due to Liver stagnation; this condition is called Liver heat toxin. Studies have determined that phenolic compounds in the plant act as antioxidants that repair liver tissue.[61] In fact, the root shows promise in treating fatty liver disease in obese individuals.[62]

While dandelion root can be an important detoxification agent for those who are discontinuing the use of opioids, it should be used only in the early stages of recovery. It can't be used long term because it is very cold in nature and can damage the digestive system (Spleen) if used for more than a month or two.

Dandelion leaves and flowers have their own medicinal properties, but the root is strongest. It tastes bitter, so most people will prefer capsules and tablets over decoctions and tinctures.

Elecampane

BOTANICAL NAME: *Inula helenium*

PARTS USED: root, flowers

DOSE: 2–4 grams daily

Elecampane fortifies the Lungs, Spleen, and Heart. It can be used therapeutically for any deficiency of the respiratory system. Elecampane can clear damp conditions of the lung and digestive tract but is not overly drying; this renders elecampane useful for varied lung conditions. It is often used in cases of chronic obstructive pulmonary disease (COPD). It also strengthens the overall immune function, and recent studies have focused on using the plant for breast and brain cancer.[63] Other studies suggest that elecampane also has anti-inflammatory qualities that could make it useful for treating conditions such as rheumatoid arthritis.[64]

Elecampane root is prepared as a decoction, but the flower, being more delicate in structure, is prepared as an infusion. Both are also often taken in the form of tinctures, capsules, or tablets.

Eleuthero (Wu Jia Pi)

BOTANICAL NAME: *Eleutherococcus senticosus*

PARTS USED: root, root bark

DOSE: 2–4 grams daily

In TCM, eleuthero is considered a warm herb that treats Kidney and Spleen yang deficiencies resulting in fatigue, sore back and knees, and poor appetite. It is also said to calm the shen and promote restful, dreamless sleep. Research suggests that its antioxidant constituents contribute to its antifatigue effects.[65] Other studies suggest that its stress-modulating effect is related to the regulation of key mediators of the stress response and the support of neurotransmitters in the brain.[66] Eleuthero is also prized for its ability to fortify the immune system.[67]

Eleuthero is commonly taken in the form of capsules, tablets, decoctions, or tinctures.

Fo-ti (He Shou Wu)

BOTANICAL NAME: *Polygonum multiflorum*

PART USED: root

DOSE: 3–6 grams daily

Fo-ti is one of the few herbs that can reinforce jing (essence); thus, it has been used as an anti-aging, anti-neurodegenerative medicine for thousands of years. Its actions are to tonify the blood, nourish the Heart, and calm the spirit. The benefits of fo-ti have been supported by scientific studies showing that antioxidant constituents in the plant help protect the organs and slow the aging process.[68]

Some studies have suggested that fo-ti can cause liver injury, but the causation remains unproven.[69] In fact, historically the herb has been used to benefit the Liver. Any damage from its use could be due to inappropriate dosing or preparation; traditionally, the roots are prepared with soybeans when used as a tonic.

Fo-ti is commonly taken in the form of capsules, tablets, decoctions, or tinctures.

Goji (Gou Qi Zi)

BOTANICAL NAME: *Lycium chinense*

PART USED: berry

DOSE: 4–8 grams daily

Goji berry is an outstanding tonic herb, nourishing the blood and reinforcing jing (essence). It is commonly used to build yin and to address patterns of Liver and Kidney deficiencies, which are common among recovering opioid users. It has a powerful effect on Lung yin energy and can help relieve coughs; it can even help restore the Lung system for ex-smokers.

Goji berry has been shown to have cardioprotective, antioxidant, anti-inflammatory properties and to moderate cholesterol levels and blood pressure.[70] Among other things, it has been shown to ameliorate many diseases common with aging, including osteoporosis,[71] and it has a long history of use with early stages of diabetes, especially in the presence of Kidney yin deficiency.

Goji berry is commonly taken in the form of capsules, tablets, decoctions, or tinctures. You can also add it to homemade energy bars and medicinal soups or just consume it out of hand as a dried fruit.

Hawthorn

BOTANICAL NAME: *Crataegus* spp.

PARTS USED: berries, leaves, flowers

DOSE: 4–8 grams daily

Hawthorn is rich in flavonoids that benefit heart health. It can normalize heart function, reduce high blood pressure, and reduce LDL cholesterol levels.[72] It takes 6 to 8 weeks for the tonic effect of hawthorn to reach any measurable level, but it is a very reliable and safe herb that can be taken long term.

The ground berries are a tasty addition to oatmeal or energy bars. Hawthorn is also commonly taken in the form of decoctions, tinctures, capsules, or tablets.

Jiao Gu Lan

BOTANICAL NAME: *Gynostemma pentaphyllum*

PART USED: leaves

DOSE: 2–4 grams daily

Jiao gu lan has a long tradition of promoting wellness and longevity among inhabitants of its natural habitat in Southeast Asia; locals regularly consume tea made from the leaves and are known to live to an old age. Jiao gu lan is considered an adaptogenic herb able to strengthen the immune response and boost the body's ability to manage stress.[73] While jiao gu lan can be used safely and for prolonged periods to improve any imbalance in the body, it is gaining popularity in its ability to moderate blood-sugar levels and stave off diabetes.[74] It can be used at any stage of diabetes and will help to correct any organ system, but recent studies have focused on its ability to protect and restore the Liver.[75] This wide range of applications shows jiao gu lan's value in helping our bodies physically adapt.

Jiao gu lan is commonly taken in the form of capsules, tablets, infusions, or tinctures.

Kratom

BOTANICAL NAME: *Mitragyna speciosa*

PART USED: leaves

DOSE: 4–6 grams three times per day

In Southeast Asia, where the plant grows, kratom has been used topically and internally for thousands of years as a fast-acting anesthetic. It was even used to combat the opium addiction crisis in Asia centuries ago.[76] It's thought that one of its constituents, mitragynine, functions as an opioid agonist, meaning that it interacts with opioid receptors in the brain. Many people use kratom not only to relieve pain but also to ease the symptoms of opioid withdrawal.

Kratom can be prepared as an infusion but is most often taken in capsule form.

Caution: Kratom is currently under review by the U.S. Drug Enforcement Agency and may at some point be classified as a controlled substance. As is the case for cannabis, the risks associated with kratom seem minuscule compared to its benefits in fighting the opioid crisis and assisting with opioid withdrawal, but be warned that more studies of kratom are needed to assess possible harmful effects of the herb. Be sure to find a reputable supplier for kratom, as its popularity has resulted in rising prices and adulterations of pure plant material. Because kratom has the potential to be misused or overused, it is recommended that it be taken only under the supervision of a health-care professional.

Lavender

BOTANICAL NAME: *Lavandula* spp.

PART USED: flowers

DOSE: 2–4 grams daily

Lavender is best known for its profound calming effect on the nervous system, but it has a plethora of medicinal applications. Promising studies have shown its benefit with anxiety, depression, and memory impairment.[77] Lavender flowers are gentle enough to use with babies yet effective enough to rid a grown person of the common cold. Lavender is cool and has a slight drying effect.

Lavender is easily prepared as an infusion, and it is also commonly taken in the form of capsules, tablets, and tinctures.

Lemon Balm

BOTANICAL NAME: *Melissa officinalis*

PART USED: leaves

DOSE: 10 grams fresh herb or 3–4 grams dried herb daily

One of few herbs gentle enough for babies, lemon balm has a calming effect while lifting the spirit and alleviating depression and anxiety.[78]

The fresh leaves are preferred because much of the healing attributes are found in the pure essential oils of this plant; dried material has lost much of the volatile oils. You can use lemon balm in a bath to help relieve stress or minor depression.

Lemon balm is most commonly taken in the form of infusions, capsules, tablets, and tinctures. The essential oil also has wonderful nervine properties, though it is quite costly.

Meadowsweet

BOTANICAL NAME: *Filipendula ulmaria*
PARTS USED: leaves, flowers
DOSE: 2–3 grams daily

Meadowsweet is effective for relieving pain; like willow bark (page 96), it contains salicin, a precursor to the salicylic acid found in aspirin, and it acts as an anti-inflammatory agent.[79] However, unlike aspirin, meadowsweet also contains tannins and other constituents that act to protect the lining of the stomach and large intestine; thus, it does not cause stomach distress.[80]

Meadowsweet makes a tasty infused tea. It can also be taken in the form of capsules, tablets, or tinctures.

Motherwort

BOTANICAL NAME: *Leonurus cardiaca*
PARTS USED: flowering tops, leaves, seeds
DOSE: 2–4 grams daily

Recent studies suggest that motherwort's cardioprotective attributes are due to its flavonoids, phenolic acids, and volatile oils, among other things.[81] Motherwort has long been used in Western herbalism to treat heart palpitations, especially when associated with menopause, and to address high blood pressure. Additionally, it is a calming nervine that can help reduce stress, depression, or anxiety that might be seen with the Kidney-Heart patterns of imbalance common in addiction recovery.[82] There are several species of motherwort that all have similar actions; the seed is favored in Chinese medicine as a blood mover for addressing pain syndromes, whereas the leaf and flowering top tend to be used in Western herbalism.

Motherwort is commonly taken in the form of infusions, tinctures, capsules, or tablets.

Caution: Motherwort is categorized as a "blood mover." It invigorates blood circulation so strongly that it must be used with caution by those who are taking blood-thinning medications or who are scheduled for surgery.

Mullein

BOTANICAL NAME: *Verbascum thapsus*
PART USED: leaves
DOSE: 3–6 grams daily

Mullein leaf is both emollient (soothing) and astringent (constricting); thus, it is able to moisten dry lungs or, conversely, clear dampness and phlegm from lungs. Mullein normalizes lung function and is able to strengthen and repair the Lung organ system, regardless of the nature of the condition. Mullein is an excellent herb for Lung qi deficiency patterns in the cases of COPD, asthma, and bronchitis.

Mullein can be prepared as an infused tea; strain the tea well, as the leaves contain tiny hairs that can irritate the lungs and throat. It is also commonly available in the form of tinctures, capsules, and tablets. You can also use the leaves topically as a poultice to relieve cramps: Pour boiling water over the leaves, and when they have cooled, apply the leaves directly to the skin, wrapped in place with a cotton cloth that has been soaked in the infused liquid.

Passionflower

BOTANICAL NAME: *Passiflora incarnata*

PARTS USED: leaves, flowers

DOSE: 2–4 grams daily

Passionflower is known for its benefits in treating anxiety, insomnia, and other symptoms of opioid withdrawal. Scientific studies have suggested that chemical constituents in the leaves of this plant bind with gabba-aminobutyric acid (GABA) receptor sites in the brain, producing the same effects as that neurotransmitter (see page 136 for more on GABA).[83] For those who have experienced brain changes due to long-term use of opioids, this is an interesting herb due to its possible ability to enhance the neuroplasticity of the brain.[84]

Passionflower leaves and flowers are often made into an infused tea that has a calming effect and may soothe nerve pain.[85] The herb is also often taken in the form of capsules, tablets, and tinctures.

Privet Fruit (Nu Zhen Zi)

BOTANICAL NAME: *Ligustrum lucidum*

PART USED: berry

DOSE: 2–4 grams daily

Privet fruit is a classic Kidney and Liver yin tonic herb that is said to prolong life. It is a significant natural immune-enhancing agent. Modern research shows that the plant increases white blood cell counts; it is used to prevent bone marrow loss in chemotherapy patients, as it contains substances that stimulate the proliferation of osteoblasts (bone-forming cells).[86] Privet fruit also contains potent antiviral qualities and antioxidants.[87]

Privet fruit is commonly consumed as a tea, though it can also be taken in the form of capsules, tablets, or tinctures.

Caution: There are many species of privet, but not all are used medicinally. Be sure you are using the *L. lucidum* species.

Red Sage (Dan Shen)

BOTANICAL NAME: *Salvia miltiorrhiza*

PART USED: root

DOSE: 1–3 grams daily

For hundreds if not thousands of years, red sage root has been used in TCM to treat heart disease. It has been shown to help repair damage after heart attacks, as well as to prevent heart disease and to repair neural cells after stroke.[88] Other promising qualities of red sage root are its ability to repair neurons in the brain that may have been damaged by opioid toxins and to improve cognitive capacity.[89] It is also known for its ability to repair liver damage.[90] It offers strong blood-moving action that can help break up the blood stagnation often associated with pain syndromes.

Red sage is commonly taken in the form of decoctions, tinctures, capsules, or tablets. It is typically used in combination with other herbs, rather than by itself.

Caution: Red sage root is categorized as a "blood mover." It invigorates blood circulation so strongly that it must be used with caution by those who are taking blood-thinning medications or who are scheduled for surgery.

Reishi (Ling Zhi)

BOTANICAL NAME: *Ganoderma lucidum*

PART USED: mushroom

DOSE: 3–6 grams daily

Reishi, a woody fungus traditionally called "the mushroom of immortality," is an immune system modulator, meaning that it normalizes immune function. Many studies have shown the benefits of reishi for cancer treatment and prevention.[91] *Shennong's Pharmacopeia*, the first known Chinese herbal text, says that "continuous consumption of reishi makes your body light and young, lengthens your life, and turns you into one like the immortal who never dies." Studies suggest that reishi's anti-aging effects are due to a lessening of oxidative stress by prolonged use of the herb.[92]

Reishi is often prepared as a decoction, but it can also be used in the form of capsules, tablets, or tinctures.

Schisandra (Wu Wei Zi)

BOTANICAL NAME: *Schisandra chinensis*

PART USED: berry

DOSE: 3–6 grams daily

Schisandra is a treasured tonic herb used in TCM to promote longevity. It has been used for generations to improve memory; studies suggest that its memory-boosting qualities are due to its ability to correct inflammatory damage done to neurons.[93] As an antioxidant, it is also showing promise in treating brain damage resulting from oxidative stress,[94] which is a common condition occurring with opioid overdose. Schisandra is one of the most useful herbs for protecting the liver and restoring liver function in cases of damage due to chemical exposure, toxins, drugs, or disease. Schisandra's hepatoprotective capabilities appear to arise from its ability to activate the enzymes that produce glutathione peroxidase, an enzyme that deactivates the free radicals that can damage liver cells.[95]

Schisandra berries are commonly taken in the form of decoctions, tinctures, capsules, or tablets.

Skullcap

BOTANICAL NAME: *Scutellaria lateriflora*

PARTS USED: leaves, flowers

DOSE: 1–3 grams daily

Skullcap is a powerful relaxant but is gentle enough to use with children. Don't confuse Western skullcap with Chinese skullcap (*Scutellaria baicalensis*), which has completely different actions; the Chinese variety clears heat, and the Western variety is the calming nervine. It is said to have a tonic effect on the nervous system when used over time and can relieve nerve spasms. This is an excellent herb for someone who is excitable or who is easily overstimulated.

Skullcap is often taken as an infusion; you can even prepare a superstrong infusion and add it to a foot bath or full-body bath to induce a peaceful night's sleep. The herb is also commonly taken in the form of capsules, tablets, or tinctures.

Turmeric

BOTANICAL NAME: *Curcuma longa*

PART USED: root

DOSE: 2–4 grams daily

Numerous studies have shown turmeric root to be a safe and effective anti-inflammatory agent.[96] While most of the research regarding turmeric has focused on its ability to lessen pain in osteoarthritis, its anti-inflammatory actions make it useful for many types of chronic inflammatory health conditions, including pain syndromes, liver imbalances, and cancer.[97]

Turmeric is typically taken in capsule form but is also available as tablets, decoctions, and tinctures. It's a common culinary spice as well, but for therapeutic purposes supplementation is advised; the amounts required to stimulate an anti-inflammatory effect may render your food distasteful.

White Peony

BOTANICAL NAME: *Paeonia laciflora*

PART USED: root

DOSE: 2–4 grams daily

White peony has a gentle, soothing nature and is highly nourishing. For this reason it has many healing applications, among them soothing the Liver, nourishing the blood, and preserving yin. It is said to break up Liver qi stagnation and is highly prized for its ability to ease both muscle cramps and the emotional disorders (such as depression, anger, and irritability) that are often seen during opioid withdrawal and recovery.[98] One of its constituents, paeoniflorin, has been shown to inhibit the growth, invasion, and metastasis of tumors.[99] Peony root is most commonly used in combination with other herbs in TCM, rather than on its own, as it can be a bit astringent, or drying, when used by itself.

Peony root is commonly taken in the form of decoctions, tinctures, capsules, or tablets.

Wild Lettuce

BOTANICAL NAME: *Lactuca virosa*

PART USED: leaves

DOSE: 1–2 grams per day

Wild lettuce's calming nervine action and pain-reducing effects make it an invaluable tool in treating opioid dependency.[100] Studies show that its potent analgesic effects may be due to the chemical constituents lactucopicrin and lactucin (a guaianolide), which bind to opioid receptor sites in the brain.[101] (Guaianolides are also found in chamomile, another gentle nervine.) One case report noted a suspicion of toxicity if the plant is taken in high doses or if the extract is injected.[102] However, there is little to no evidence that the plant is toxic if consumed in doses traditionally prescribed in herbal medicine.

Wild lettuce can be infused as a tea, but it is bitter. It is also commonly taken in capsule, tablet, or tincture forms. The very young shoots of the wild plant are often steamed and added to dishes as you would spinach, but again, the taste can be a bit bitter.

Willow

BOTANICAL NAME: *Salix alba*
PART USED: bark
DOSE: 1–3 grams daily

Like meadowsweet (page 89), willow bark contains salicin, a precursor to the salicylic acid found in aspirin, and it acts as an anti-inflammatory agent. It is a powerful and effective pain reliever. There are around 400 species of willow; all contain salicin.

Willow is taken in the form of decoctions or capsules.

Yarrow

BOTANICAL NAME: *Achillea millefolium*
PARTS USED: leaves, flowers
DOSE: 2–3 grams daily

A traditional European remedy, yarrow has been used to reduce pain since ancient times. TCM classifies it as a "blood mover," and it is said to break up blood stagnation that leads to pain. A few recent studies have shown the value of this humble herb in pain relief when used both topically and internally.[103]

Yarrow makes a nice infused tea, but can also be taken in capsule, tablet, or tincture form. It can also be applied topically to relieve pain: Pour boiling water over the leaves, cover, and let cool. Then apply the leaves directly on the skin over the painful areas, and wrap them in place with a strip of cotton cloth that has been soaked in the infused tea.

Yellow Dock

BOTANICAL NAME: *Rumex crispus*

PART USED: root

DOSE: 2–4 grams daily

Yellow dock has a long tradition as a liver-cleansing herb. The bitter compounds can also stimulate a cascade effect on the digestive system and help gently resolve opioid-related constipation. It is a rich source of iron and is considered a blood cleanser and builder. It has also been suggested that yellow dock has powerful antioxidant qualities and is able to repair damage from toxins.[104] While a gentle remedy, yellow dock is effective at clearing Liver heat, or toxins, for those who have been using opioids; this can help with opioid-induced itchiness.

Yellow dock root tastes bitter, so most people will prefer capsules and tablets over decoctions and tinctures.

CHAPTER 5

Essential Oils and Flower Essences
Therapeutic Support for the Body and Spirit

Essential oils are highly aromatic and volatile plant constituents that are most often extracted by steam distillation. The distillation process makes them potent, which means that you need only a small amount to have the desired effect. Herbs contain many other types of active ingredients besides essential oils; therefore, the actions of essential oils may vary somewhat from the actions of herbal medicines made from the whole plant. It takes a great deal of plant material to extract small amounts of essential oils, and that's one reason they are so costly.

Essential oils resemble vegetable oils in the fact that they are not water soluble; however, they are distinct from vegetable oils in that they are made up of esters and have a high evaporation rate, especially when exposed to heat. Therefore, they are sometimes referred to as "volatile oils."

For the purposes of this book, we are focused on using essential oils to balance the five elements of Chinese medicine (Water, Wood, Fire, Earth, Metal) and thus stimulate healthy qi flow, yin-yang balance, emotional balance, and normalized physical function in an effort to help opioid users through the period of withdrawal and recovery. To that end, the profiles in this section will detail which acupressure points you can apply each essential oil to in order to target the stimulation of a particular element and/or organ system. There are, of course, many other ways to use essential oils, particularly in aromatherapy, but we'll leave that discussion for another book.

Carrier Oils

Carrier oils are vegetable and nut oils used to dilute essential oils. Most essential oils are too concentrated to be applied undiluted, or neat, to the skin. Unless otherwise indicated, they should be diluted in a carrier oil at a concentration of about 6 to 10 percent. (That's roughly 1 to 2 drops of essential oil in 1 teaspoon of carrier oil.) Here are a few carrier oils to consider:

- Olive oil is an ideal carrier oil because it does not become rancid as quickly as other oils. Traditionally, the first press of olive oil (virgin oil) is used for cooking and the second press is used in cosmetics and healing remedies. The second-press oil is less expensive and has the added benefit of having a less pungent odor.

- Grapeseed oil is odor free and, like olive oil, very stable, so it will not spoil quickly.

- Almond oil is a very light oil that is easily absorbed by your skin. It contains vitamins, including A, B, and E, and nourishes the skin. It has a slight nutty aroma.

- Coconut oil comes in both refined and unrefined versions. For use with essential oils you will want the refined oil, as it is in a liquid rather than a solid state. It does smell like coconut, so only use this oil if you find that odor appealing.

ELEMENTAL INFLUENCES OF ESSENTIAL OILS

ELEMENT	ESSENTIAL OILS TO ACTIVATE THIS ELEMENT		
WATER	basil	fennel	nutmeg
	cedar	geranium	rosemary
	cinnamon leaf	ginger	thyme
	clary sage	lavender	
	clove	marjoram	
WOOD	anise seed	fennel	lavender
	citrus (qing pi)	frankincense	marjoram
	clary sage	ho wood	rosemary
FIRE	cinnamon leaf	geranium	lavender
	clary sage	ginger	marjoram
	cypress	ho wood	rosemary
	frankincense		
EARTH	anise seed	clove	geranium
	basil	coriander	ginger
	cinnamon leaf	cypress	ho wood
	citrus (qing pi and chen pi)	eucalyptus	marjoram
		fennel	nutmeg
	clary sage	frankincense	rosemary
METAL	anise seed	citrus (chen pi)	ginger
	basil	clary sage	nutmeg
	cedar	cypress	thyme
	cinnamon leaf	eucalyptus	

Essential Oils: Profiles

The essential oils listed below are those that I would consider most beneficial for people who are in the stages of withdrawal and recovery from opioid use. The profiles note which elements each essential oil can reinforce and the indications for their use.

All of the acupuncture points mentioned in these profiles can be found in the illustrated guide beginning on page 62.

Anise Seed

BOTANICAL NAME: *Pimpinella anisum*
ELEMENTAL ASSOCIATIONS: Wood, Earth, Metal
CORRELATING ORGAN SYSTEMS: Liver, Spleen, Stomach, Lungs
NATURE: warm, sweet, spicy, drying

Indications for Use

To reinforce Wood: Soothes the Liver and breaks up qi stagnation that results in restlessness, frustration, emotional upset, and stress. Liver qi stagnation, if left untreated, turns to Liver heat, which can result in insomnia. Can be diluted and applied topically over the ribs/liver. Apply to acupoints LV 2 and LV 3.

To reinforce Earth: Helps calm spasms that result in relentless hiccups (often seen with opioid withdrawal) and resolves nausea, stomach cramps, and vomiting of clear fluids. Can be rubbed on the abdomen for indigestion such as spasms, pain, and stomach upset. Apply to acupoints SP 3, SP 9, ST 36, and CV 12.

To reinforce Metal: Used to reinforce Lung qi and tonify qi in cases of deficiency due to stress and overwork. Also dries respiratory phlegm and stops persistent spasmodic coughing seen in opioid cessation. Can be diluted and applied topically over the chest and upper back. Apply to acupoints LU 5, LU 7, and LU 9.

Basil

BOTANICAL NAME: *Ocimum basilicum*
ELEMENTAL ASSOCIATIONS: Water, Earth, Metal
CORRELATING ORGAN SYSTEMS: Kidneys, Spleen, Stomach, Lungs
NATURE: warm, sweet, spicy, drying

Indications for Use

To reinforce Water: Sweet basil impacts the adrenal cortex and the brain, enhancing cognition and aiding with exhaustion and muddled thinking following opioid use. Reinforces Kidney qi and Kidney yang, thus restoring vitality after chronic exhaustion results in adrenal fatigue and/or nervous depression. Use as a Kidney yang tonic with chronic lower back pain and achiness of the knees. Apply to the lower back over the kidneys for Kidney yang deficiency. Apply to acupoints KI 3, KI 6, and CV 6.

To reinforce Earth: Applied to the stomach to address indigestion, poor digestion of meats and fats, and abdominal distention. Best used for these conditions when applying heat to the abdomen improves the stomach upset or pain. Used for nausea and poor appetite related to opioid withdrawal. Apply to acupoints SP 3, ST 36, and CV 12.

To reinforce Metal: Breaks up feelings of chest tightness (lungs) and wheezing. Dries phlegm and expectorates phlegm from the lungs; this may result in more coughing, which can be undesirable after stopping opioids. Fresh juice extracted from basil leaves is more effective at stopping coughs than the essential oil is. Can be applied topically over the chest and upper back. Apply to acupoints LU 5, LU 7, and LU 9.

Cedar

BOTANICAL NAME: *Cedrus deodara*

ELEMENTAL ASSOCIATIONS: Water, Metal

CORRELATING ORGAN SYSTEMS: Bladder, Lungs

NATURE: cool, spicy

Indications for Use

To reinforce Water: Drains damp heat in the pelvic area, which would include painful burning urination or vaginal discharge with foul odor. Apply directly to abdomen and to acupoints BL 62 and SI 3.

To reinforce Metal: Improves breathing and opens the chest. Can be applied topically over the chest and upper back for improved breathing. Apply along the Lung channel for pain and swelling, especially in the wrist, elbow, and shoulder joints. Apply to acupoints LU 5, LU 7, and LU 9.

Cinnamon Leaf

BOTANICAL NAME: *Cinnamomum cassia*

ELEMENTAL ASSOCIATIONS: Water, Fire, Earth, Metal

CORRELATING ORGAN SYSTEMS: Bladder, Heart, Lungs

NATURE: hot, spicy, sweet

Indications for Use

To reinforce Water: Anchors and stimulates the movement of yang; anchors the yang to prevent dispersion; for Kidney yang deficiency, coldness, and adrenal exhaustion. Apply to the lower back over the kidneys and at acupoints KI 3 and CV 6.

To reinforce Fire: Used to break up stagnation in the chest due to cold and resulting in sharp pain, palpitations, and poor circulation. Apply to extremities to improve blood circulation. Apply directly over the chest and at acupoints HT 7, PER 6, and PER 7.

To reinforce Earth: Because cinnamon is hot, it can work to resolve pain syndromes related to cold and internal dampness. Apply to the abdomen for stomach pain and upset relieved by warmth. Apply over areas of muscle and joint pain that are improved with the application of warmth, because cinnamon acts as an anti-inflammatory.[105] For feelings of pain with heaviness, apply to acupoint SP 9.

To reinforce Metal: Used to relieve pain along the Lung channel due to cold or damp, especially shoulder pain. Apply directly to the channel and at acupoints LU 5, LU 7, and LU 9.

Clary Sage

BOTANICAL NAME: *Salvia sclarea*
ELEMENTAL ASSOCIATIONS: Water, Wood, Fire, Earth, Metal
CORRELATING ORGAN SYSTEMS: Liver, Heart, Kidneys
NATURE: warm/neutral, spicy, sweet

Indications for Use

To reinforce Water: Addresses Kidney qi and Yin deficiency with symptoms such as anxiety, panic attacks, hot flashes, afternoon sweats, and night sweats. Apply to acupoint KI 3.

To reinforce Wood: Soothes the Liver, subdues Liver heat resulting in internal wind, thus subduing spasms such as the leg spasms seen during opioid detox. Apply to muscles affected by spasms, along the ribs, and at acupoints LV 2, LV 3, GB 34, and GB 41.

To reinforce Fire: Calms the shen when there is insomnia, emotional tension, and headaches. Has a calming effect on the mind, but revives poor cognition. Restores clarity following chronic stress resulting in exhaustion, as is experienced after opioid cessation. Apply to acupoints HT 7, PER 6, and PER 7.

To reinforce Earth: Used for stomach upset due to nervous tension. Apply to acupoints SP 3, SP 6, and ST 36.

To reinforce Metal: Opens the chest during withdrawal for those with shortness of breath and the feeling of chest/lung compression experienced during withdrawal and in the months thereafter. Apply over the upper chest and upper back and at acupoints KI 6, LU 5, LU 7, and LU 9.

Clove

BOTANICAL NAME: *Eugenia caryophyllata*

ELEMENTAL ASSOCIATIONS: Water, Earth

CORRELATING ORGAN SYSTEMS: Kidneys, Spleen, Stomach

NATURE: warm, spicy

Indications for Use

To reinforce Water: Used to reinforce the Kidney yang seen with symptoms of coldness in the body or legs and hands, weakness of legs or knees, chronic lower back pain, or adrenal exhaustion. Improves cognition after a long period of depletion and fatigue. Apply to the lower back over the kidneys and at acupoints KI 3 and CV 6.

To reinforce Earth: Warms the middle in cases of vomiting, nausea, abdominal pain/spasms, and lack of appetite due to cold. Use topically for pain as an anti-inflammatory[106] or in pain conditions that improve with heat. Apply directly onto the abdomen and at acupoints SP 3, SP 6, and ST 36.

Coriander

BOTANICAL NAME: *Coriandrum sativum*

ELEMENTAL ASSOCIATIONS: Earth

CORRELATING ORGAN SYSTEMS: Spleen, Stomach, Lungs

NATURE: warm, sweet, spicy

Indications for Use

To reinforce Earth: Reinforces Spleen qi with deficient indications such as lack of appetite, loose stools, poor digestion, and nausea. Dispels internal dampness and pain syndromes due to dampness impeding qi flow in the channels with a feeling of heavy limbs. Used to calm stomach upset, cramping, and spasms. Helpful when a prolonged period of neglect results in deficiency, depression, slow cognition, and foggy brain. Use topically for pain related to dampness. Apply directly onto the abdomen and at acupoints SP 3, SP 6, SP 9, and ST 36.

Cypress

BOTANICAL NAME: *Cupressus sempervirens*

ELEMENTAL ASSOCIATIONS: Fire, Earth, Metal

CORRELATING ORGAN SYSTEMS: Spleen, Lungs

NATURE: slightly cool, dry, spicy, sweet

Indications for Use

To reinforce Fire: Stimulates blood circulation. Apply directly to limbs, hands, and feet.

To reinforce Earth: Breaks up lymph fluid congestion. Dries dampness. Assists with nausea. Apply over lymph-rich areas and to acupoints PER 6, SP 3, SP 6, and SP 9.

To reinforce Metal: Soothes spasmatic coughing, clears Lung phlegm and infections, and addresses asthma with difficulty inhaling. Astringes the skin and promotes tissue healing; removes toxic heat of the skin, as seen with red rashes and boils originating from blood heat. Apply to inflamed skin, to the upper chest over the lungs, and to acupoints KI 6, LU 5, LU 7, LU 9, and LI 11.

Eucalyptus

BOTANICAL NAME: *Eucalyptus globulus*

ELEMENTAL ASSOCIATIONS: Earth, Metal

CORRELATING ORGAN SYSTEMS: Spleen, Lungs

NATURE: warm, spicy

Indications for Use

To reinforce Earth: Applied to painful, swollen joints and muscles that worsen in damp weather. Apply over affected areas.

To reinforce Metal: Clears phlegm from the respiratory system, including sinuses and lungs. Apply over affected areas.

Fennel

BOTANICAL NAME: *Foeniculum vulgare*
ELEMENTAL ASSOCIATIONS: Water, Wood, Earth
CORRELATING ORGAN SYSTEMS: Kidneys, Liver, Spleen, Stomach
NATURE: warm, spicy, sweet

Indications for Use

To reinforce Water: Warms the Kidneys and tonifies Kidney qi. Reinforces the Bladder qi in cases of incontinence or frequent urinary tract infections. Apply to the lower back over the kidneys and to acupoints KI 3, KI 6, BL 60, BL 62, and LU 7.

To reinforce Wood: Apply along the Liver channel in cases of pain that improves with warmth. Apply to acupoints LV 2, LV 3, and GB 34.

To reinforce Earth: Promotes digestion and absorption of nutrients. Resolves phlegm and coughing that produces clear or white phlegm. Warms the Stomach for those with stomach upset, abdominal pain, poor digestion of meats and fats, nausea, or vomiting that is resolved when warmth is applied over the stomach. Apply to the abdomen and at acupoints SP 3, SP 6, SP 9, and ST 36. For coughs, apply over the upper chest and upper back and to acupoints KI 6 and LU 7.

Frankincense

BOTANICAL NAME: *Boswellia carterii*
ELEMENTAL ASSOCIATIONS: Wood, Fire, Earth
CORRELATING ORGAN SYSTEMS: Liver, Heart, Spleen
NATURE: warm, spicy

Indications for Use

To reinforce Wood: Used as an ingredient in remedies to treat pain from internal wind with spasms. Enhances the Liver's ability to promote the free flow of qi throughout the body and opens the diaphragm for better breathing. Apply to areas of pain and to acupoints LV 2, LV 3, GB 34, GB 41, and LI 4.

To reinforce Fire: Promotes blood flow and breaking up blood and qi stagnation associated with pain and swelling. Calms the shen when emotional upset and sleep disturbances are present. Apply to the chest to ease Heart blood congestion and sharp pain. (But of course you should call 911 if you suspect a heart attack.) Apply to areas of pain and to acupoints LV 3, HT 7, and LI 4.

To reinforce Earth: Used as a remedy for "damp bi" (*bi* simply means pain), or internal dampness restricting the flow of blood and qi and resulting in pain. Enhances the Spleen's ability to regenerate flesh for wounds and scars. Apply to skin or areas of pain and to acupoints LV 3, LI 4, SP 3, SP 6, and SP 9.

Geranium

BOTANICAL NAME: *Pelargonium graveolens*
ELEMENTAL ASSOCIATIONS: Water, Fire, Earth
CORRELATING ORGAN SYSTEMS: Kidneys, Heart, Conception Vessel
NATURE: cool, sweet

Indications for Use

To reinforce Water: Addresses Kidney yin deficiency with symptoms such as night sweats and night terrors during withdrawal and long-term adrenal fatigue. Also used for trouble taking a deep breath following cessation of opioid use. Apply to acupoints KI 3, KI 6, HT 7, LU 7, and CV 6.

To reinforce Fire: Calms the shen with emotional disturbances and sleep issues. Helps to circulate blood and qi to relieve pain, spasms, and inflammation. Apply over areas of pain and to acupoints HT 7, HT 8, PER 6, PER 7, SP 4, ST 36, and CV 6.

To reinforce Earth: Used to help even out blood-sugar levels after opioid use. Apply over areas of dense lymph nodes to help with detoxification during opioid withdrawal. Apply to acupoints SP 3, SP 6, ST 36, and CV 12.

Ginger

BOTANICAL NAME: *Zingiber officinale*
ELEMENTAL ASSOCIATIONS: Water, Fire, Earth, Metal
CORRELATING ORGAN SYSTEMS: Heart, Spleen, Stomach, Lungs
NATURE: hot, spicy

Note: For this application, look for ginger essential oil that was extracted from the dried root, rather than the fresh root.

Indications for Use

To reinforce Water: Rescues devastated yang with indications of prolonged feeling of coldness throughout the body. Apply to the lower back over the kidneys and to acupoints KI 3, KI 6, LU 7, and CV 6.

To reinforce Fire: Invigorates blood, warms the channels, and increases circulation. For any pain that improves with the application of heat, but especially muscular pain that worsens with damp weather and/or cold weather. Apply to limbs and/or over areas of pain and to acupoints LV 3, ST 36, and LI 4.

To reinforce Earth: For those with nausea, vomiting of clear fluids, a thirst for warm drinks, and cold limbs. Use for indigestion and stomach upset that is improved with heat. Revives Spleen yang with indications of loose stools and poor appetite, and wei qi (immunity) for recovering addicts who have had prolonged nutritional deficiencies. Apply to the abdomen and at acupoints KI 3, SP 3, SP 6, SP 9, ST 36, and CV 6.

To reinforce Metal: Used to restore Lung yang with indications of chronic runny nose and/or slight coughs with clear, white, or foamy sputum. For pale asthmatics and fully depleted opioid survivors who have trouble breathing. Apply to the upper chest and back over the lungs and to acupoints KI 6, LU 5, LU 7, LU 9, and CV 6.

Ho Wood

BOTANICAL NAME: *Cinnamomum camphora*
(ho-shu variety, not to be confused with white camphor)
ELEMENTAL ASSOCIATIONS: Wood, Fire, Earth
CORRELATING ORGAN SYSTEMS: Liver, Heart, Spleen
NATURE: warm, floral, sweet, pungent

Indications for Use

To reinforce Wood: Soothes the Liver and treats Liver qi rising, resulting in headaches and migraines. Supports the Liver in its ability to circulate qi freely throughout the body thus helping to relieve muscle and joint pain due to qi stagnation as well as muscle spasms due to internal wind. Apply to acupoints LV 2, LV 3, GB 34, GB 41, and LI 4.

To reinforce Fire: Calms the shen when nervous tension and exhaustive nervous depression are present. Helps to reestablish emotional warmth following interpersonal divisions due to opioid use. Apply to acupoints KI 3, HT 7, PER 7, LU 9, and CV 6.

To reinforce Earth: Assists the Spleen function of regenerating flesh as it is applied to cuts for speedy healing and scar reduction. Has rejuvenating and restorative qi tonic-type actions. Apply directly to skin and/or to acupoints SP 3, SP 6, ST 36, and CV 6.

Lavender

BOTANICAL NAME: *Lavandula* spp.
ELEMENTAL ASSOCIATIONS: Water, Wood, Fire
CORRELATING ORGAN SYSTEMS: Kidney, Liver, Heart
NATURE: cool, bit dry

Indications for Use

To reinforce Water: Helps to calm anxiety. Apply to acupoints KI 3, KI 6, and HT 5.

To reinforce Wood: Breaks up Liver qi stagnation with indications of agitation, depression, and headaches. Apply to acupoints LV 2, LV 3,

GB 34, and GB 41. Combine with ho wood essential oil and apply to acupoint GB 1 for headaches at the temples.

To reinforce Fire: Calms the shen with emotional upset and sleep disturbances. Calms heart palpitations and promotes blood circulation. Restores calm focus in those who have suffered cognitive impairment due to opioid use. Apply to acupoints HT 7, HT 8, PER 6, PER 7, and PER 8.

Mandarin Orange/Tangerine
BOTANICAL NAME: *Citrus reticulata*
ELEMENTAL ASSOCIATIONS: green peel — Wood, Earth
mature peel — Earth, Metal
CORRELATING ORGAN SYSTEMS: green peel — Liver, Gallbladder, Stomach
mature peel — Spleen, Stomach, Lungs
NATURE: bitter, spicy, warm

Note: The essential oil derived from the green peel (qing pi) and that derived from the mature peel (chen pi) have different indications for use.

Indications for Use: Qing Pi (Green Peel)
To reinforce Wood: Breaks up Liver qi stagnation with indications such as headaches, premenstrual syndrome (PMS), anger, frustration, and aggression. Apply directly over the liver at the lower portion of the ribs and at acupoints LV 2 and LV 3.

To reinforce Earth: Used to break up accumulations and stagnation of undigested food. Resolves dampness. Apply directly to the abdomen and at acupoints SP 3, SP 6, SP 9, and ST 36.

Indications for Use: Chen Pi (Mature Peel)
To reinforce Earth: Improves the function of the Spleen, including absorption of nutrients from food. Resolves internal dampness associated with Spleen qi deficiency. Apply anywhere along the Spleen channel to break up stagnation resulting in pain. Apply directly on the abdomen and at acupoints SP 3, SP 6, SP 9, and ST 36.

To reinforce Metal: Resolves phlegm in the lungs and sinuses. Breaks up qi stagnation along the Lung channel resulting in pain. Apply anywhere along the Lung channel for pain. Apply directly on chest over the lungs and at acupoints SP 9, LU 5, LU 7, and LU 9.

Marjoram

BOTANICAL NAME: *Origanum majorana*
ELEMENTAL ASSOCIATIONS: Water, Wood, Fire, Earth
CORRELATING ORGAN SYSTEMS: Kidneys, Liver, Heart, Spleen
NATURE: cool, pungent, sweet, a bit drying

Indications for Use

To reinforce Water: Reinforces Kidney yin and jing, and is used to heal brain function and improve memory and cognition for those who have been using opioids for an extended period. Apply to acupoints KI 3, KI 6, and CV 6.

To reinforce Wood: Soothes the Liver and quenches Liver fire with agitation and aggressiveness. Descends Liver fire rising that results in headaches and migraines. Resolves internal wind due to Liver fire that results in twitches and spasms (experienced commonly during detox), but addresses most any condition with muscle spasms. Works as an uplifting remedy for nervous exhaustion. Apply directly to spasmotic areas and to acupoints LV 2, LV 3, GB 34, GB 40, GB 41, and LI 4.

To reinforce Fire: Calms the shen when emotional nervousness, upset, frustration, and sleep disturbances with vivid dreams are present. Strengthens the Heart and encourages the circulation of Heart qi and blood. Apply to acupoints HT 7, HT 8, PER 7, and PER 8.

To reinforce Earth: Calms digestive upset and acid reflux. Resolves internal dampness resulting in pain syndromes, especially in swollen red joints that worsen in damp conditions; hot, humid climates; and periods of rain. Apply at sites of pain and at acupoints SP 3, SP 6, SP 9, ST 36, and CV 12.

Nutmeg

BOTANICAL NAME: *Myristica fragrans*
ELEMENTAL ASSOCIATIONS: Water, Earth, Metal
CORRELATING ORGAN SYSTEMS: Liver, Spleen, Stomach
NATURE: Warm, spicy

Indications for Use

To reinforce Water: Apply to lower back over kidneys. In cases of yang deficiency, apply at acupoints KI 3 and CV 6.

To reinforce Earth: Used to treat diarrhea and abdominal pain and distention that improves when heat is applied. Apply to the lower abdomen. For pain in the extremities due to internal dampness blocking the free flow of qi and blood with feelings of heaviness, apply directly to the extremities and/or joints. Also apply to acupoints SP 3, SP 9, ST 36, and CV 12.

To reinforce Metal: Apply to the chest and to acupoints LU 5, LU 7, and LU 9 for chronic coughing. For pain along the Large Intestine channel of the hand, arms, elbow, and shoulder, apply directly to these areas and at acupoint LI 4.

Rosemary

BOTANICAL NAME: *Rosmarinus officinalis*
ELEMENTAL ASSOCIATIONS: Water, Wood, Fire, Earth
CORRELATING ORGAN SYSTEMS: Kidney, Liver, Heart, Spleen
NATURE: warm spicy, sweet, dry

Indications for Use

To reinforce Water: Used to reinforce the adrenal cortex. Also used to improve memory, concentration, and cognition. Apply to acupoints KI 3, KI 6, HT 7, and CV 6.

To reinforce Wood: Restores the nervous system and calms emotional nervous tension, headaches, and migraines. Relieves joint pain, and spasms in the muscles. Apply directly to areas of pain and at acupoints LV 2, LV 3, and GB 41.

To reinforce Fire: Serves as a heart tonic and a blood circulation tonic. Apply to limbs to increase circulation and to acupoints HT 7 and PER 7.

To reinforce Earth: Used to treat chronic diarrhea with mucus in the stools. Apply to acupoints SP 3, SP 6, SP 9, and ST 36.

Thyme

BOTANICAL NAME: *Thymus vulgaris*

ELEMENTAL ASSOCIATIONS: Water, Metal

CORRELATING ORGAN SYSTEMS: Kidneys, Lungs

NATURE: warm, spicy, sweet, drying

Indications for Use

To reinforce Water: Improves memory, concentration, and cognition in cases of brain function decline. Reinforces adrenal cortex for fatigue due to adrenal exhaustion. Apply to acupoints KI 3, KI 6, and LU 7.

To reinforce Metal: Used to treat coughs with phlegm. Apply over the upper chest and upper back and to acupoints LU 5, LU 7, and LU 9.

Flower Essences: Profiles

Flower essences are made by infusing water with fresh flowers in sunlight. You can make them yourself at home (you can find instructions online and in various books on herbal medicine), but most people buy them.

Like acupuncture, flower essences are a subtle energy medicine, but they work on an even higher vibrational level than herbs and essential oils. In fact, you can use flower essences to enhance the effects of other botanical remedies and natural healing modalities. You can apply them to specific acupoints, like essential oils, or you can spritz them over your body or in your environment. In general, flower essences are used therapeutically to clear deep emotional issues and support mind-body wellness. They strengthen our abilities to work through personal challenges and overcome obstacles that block us from living life to our fullest potential — and that is why they are so wonderful as remedies to facilitate recovery from opioid dependency.

One 2017 study suggested that people with anxiety and depression consume a disproportionate share of prescription painkillers like opioids. In the early stages of the U.S. opioid epidemic, authorities routinely stated that addiction to prescription opioids begins with some physical ailment that causes pain for which an opioid is prescribed. This narrative rarely considered the mental health of such patients. It now is understood that people suffering from depression and other mental health disorders are more susceptible to opioid-induced euphoria and can become dependent on the drugs more quickly.[107] Flower essences can play an important role in clearing emotional pain for people who are struggling with opioid dependence, including those with mental health disorders.

Flower essences were discovered in the 1930s by Edward Bach, an English homeopathic doctor, and therefore they are sometimes called Bach flower remedies. The flower essences listed here are those I would consider most beneficial for people who are in the stages of withdrawal and recovery from opioid use.

Agrimony

The flower essence agrimony benefits the Fire element and allows the Pericardium, or Heart protector, to heal from life's emotional insults. The Pericardium is said to function as a gate that, when open, allows us to accept joy and love. Agrimony helps those who try to hide their negative emotions behind the Pericardium and who only feel happiness when intoxicated. It also helps to release inner tensions and is used with anxiety disorders and post-traumatic stress disorder (PTSD). Dr. Bach noted that those who would benefit from the remedy "often take alcohol or drugs in excess, to stimulate themselves and help themselves bear their trials with cheerfulness."[108] Agrimony aids those who are tortured by unpleasant memories and emotions that have been suppressed behind drug use and have resurfaced with the discontinuation of opioids.

Cherry Plum

The flower essence of cherry plum allows us to reconnect to our true karmic path and bolsters our ability to follow our own inner guidance. This remedy allows us to let go and accept higher guidance. Cherry plum can help resolve the fear of losing control that sometimes accompanies addiction, and it helps us face extreme hardship with equanimity. This remedy can aid those experiencing extreme dark emotions, such as thoughts of suicide or believing they are about to lose their mind.

Chestnut Bud

Chestnut bud flower essence helps us break the cycle of making the wrong choice over and over again. It can help people with opioid addiction avoid repeating the bad decisions that keep them stuck in the cycle of addiction. Chestnut bud also helps us develop skills of observation and listening, allowing us to gain life lessons from others' mistakes and examples rather than having to learn only from personal experience. It can help us recognize patterns of behavior that lead to poor outcomes. This ability to understand cause and effect better allows those in recovery to avoid the environmental triggers that lead to cravings and opioid use.

Walnut

Dr. Bach called walnut flower essence the "breaker of spells" for its ability to dissolve the bonds that hold us to past events and to past addictive behaviors.[109] It allows for a transition away from the influence of others and their opinions so that those in recovery are able to return to their true path. Walnut also helps protect us against outside influences and the impact of life's inevitable changes, such as moving, changing jobs, or losing a loved one.

Wild Rose

Wild rose flower essence restores the shen (spirit) and restores a love of life and sense of purpose following a long struggle resulting in exhaustion. Wild rose restores to us a vision for a better life while allowing us to discard apathetic beliefs that things will never change.

Flower Essence Blend for Opioid Recovery

Flower essences, when combined, have a synergistic effect. In other words, the combined remedy has a greater therapeutic effect than taking every essence individually. Spray the remedy on wrists, neck, and/or appropriate acupoints described on the following pages.

INGREDIENTS

- 3 tablespoons distilled water
- 1 teaspoon brandy
- 10 drops agrimony flower essence
- 10 drops cherry plum flower essence
- 10 drops chestnut bud flower essence
- 10 drops walnut flower essence
- 10 drops wild rose flower essence

PREPARATION

Pour the water and brandy into a 2-ounce glass bottle with a spritzer top and shake to mix. Add the flower essences. Shake the bottle for 30 seconds. Shake again before each application.

Using Flower Essences with Acupoints

Certain acupuncture/acupressure points have profound impacts on shen. These points work to restore harmony on a psycho-emotional level. Since flower essences operate on that same vibrational level and interact with shen, they can have a powerful effect when applied to those points.

To ease withdrawal and facilitate recovery from opioids, I recommend applying all of the flower essences listed previously as a blend from a spritzer bottle (see page 117). The acupoints that are most beneficial for use with flower essences are listed below, and they all happen to fall on the wrists, chest, and abdomen. With a few spritzes from the bottle, you can thus quickly and easily apply healing flower essences to all of the points several times a day. If you have the time and inclination, you can then follow up with acupressure on the points (see chapter 3) to reinforce the flower essences' energy.

I list the acupoints below with a translation of their original ancient Chinese names, because the names often coincide with the intention of the points' application.

All of these points can be found in the illustrated guide beginning on page 62.

Acupoints on the Abdomen

CV 8 *TCM name:* Spirit Deficiency
Location: At the center of the belly button.

Drug use dulls shen (spirit), leading to a disconnection from your true self. This point reestablishes communication between the body and the spirit, thus grounding the mind. It can be especially helpful in cases of mental instability.

KI 16 *TCM name:* Vital Correspondence
Location: 0.5 cun on either side of the belly button.

This point is a link between shen and jing (essence), opening the way for shen to be nourished and linked to our ancestral qi and karmic path.

KI 20 and K 21 *TCM names:* Through the Valley and Dark Gate

Location: KI 20 is found on the upper abdomen, 5 cun above the center of the belly button and 0.5 cun lateral to the anterior midline; KI 21 is also on the upper abdomen, 6 cun above the center of the belly button and 0.5 cun lateral to the anterior midline.

KI 20 and KI 21 are paired acupoints that allow transformational passage through the darkness and negativity of depression into the light of self-actualization and peace of mind.

Acupoints on the Chest

CV 17 *TCM name:* Central Altar
Location: On the anterior median line of the chest, at the level of the fourth intercostal space (the space between the ribs); for men, this is at the midpoint between the two nipples.

CV 17 is indicated with any Fire element imbalance. It calms shen disturbances such as emotional upset. Used to reestablish one's rightful placement between heaven and earth, allowing for a sense of belonging.

CV 20 *TCM name:* Floral Covering
Location: On the anterior median line of the chest, at the level of the first intercostal space.

Allows one to bloom into full fruition, bursting into the sunlight of recovery.

KI 22 *TCM name:* Walking the Corridor
Location: On the chest, in the depression in the fifth intercostal space, 2 cun lateral to the anterior midline.

Assists in the progressive walk away from fear and the emergence at a place of peace and joy.

KI 23 *TCM name:* Spirit Seal
Location: On the chest, in the depression in the fourth intercostal space, 2 cun lateral to the anterior midline.

Like the seal on an envelope, the Spirit Seal is a personal mark of identity. This acupoint fosters the ability to emerge from the despair of addiction and rediscover one's true self.

KI 24 *TCM name:* Spirit Ruins or Spirit Burial Ground
Location: On the chest, in the depression in the third intercostal space, 2 cun lateral to the anterior midline.

Allows one to escape from the darkness of a tomb of despair and depression, and to emerge into a bright light of happiness and self-fulfillment.

KI 25 *TCM name:* Spirit Storehouse
Location: On the chest, in the depression in the second intercostal space, 2 cun lateral to the anterior midline.

We are born with ancestral jing that is stored in the Kidneys. When chronic opioid use exhausts our jing, we become fearful and fall into despair. This point helps us reestablish our access to the Water element, replenishing the original essence so that we can proceed fearlessly into recovery.

KI 26 *TCM name:* Flourishing Center or Lively Center
Location: On the chest, in the depression in the first intercostal space, 2 cun lateral to the anterior midline.

This point is used to allow the qi of the chest to circulate smoothly. This is where the Heart resides; it is the center of the emotions. With the smooth flow of qi to the Heart, the shen brightly shines through and restores a lively childlike joy to life. With the Fire element in balance, the emotions are normalized and we can flourish.

KI 27
TCM name: Transport Treasure
Location: On the chest, in the depression on the lower border of the clavicle, 2 cun lateral to the anterior midline.

The highest spirit point, and the last point on the Kidney channel, this is the point of arrival. The qi of the Kidney energetic stream flows to this point. Here is the palace or mansion of all our highest faculties, which have been conferred on us by the Kidney energetic system.

Acupoints on the Wrist

PER 6
TCM name: Inner Passage
Location: On the palm side of the forearm, 2 cun above the crease of the wrist between the tendons of the palmaris longus muscle and the flexor carpi radialis muscle.

The Pericardium is the door to the Heart; it opens to allow love in, and closes to keep emotional hurts out. When damaged, it can remain stuck closed. The Heart is the only organ that is assigned another organ for its protection. This is because the Heart houses the emotions, and damage to the Heart creates mental disorders and emotional chaos. This point is used to allow us to acknowledge the damage that opioid use has created, while healing the Pericardium. It allows for us to open our Heart and reunite with loved ones following the destruction of personal relationships due to opioid dependency.

PER 7
TCM name: Great Mound
Location: On the palm side of the crease of the wrist dividing the arm from the hand between the tendons of the palmaris longus muscle and the flexor carpi radialis muscle.

A mound is a pile of earth, and acupoint PER 7 is the Earth point on a Fire element channel. It is used to ground our emotions after flying high on euphoria-inducing opioids. This euphoric condition can be compared to mania, which in TCM is a hyper-yang state with Heart fire. PER 7 clears heat from the Heart and calms the extreme emotional outbursts seen during withdrawal of opioids.

HT 5
TCM name: Penetrating Inside
Location: On the inside of the wrist, on the radial side of the tendon of the flexor carpi ulnaris muscle, 1 cun above the crease of the wrist.

In TCM, the Heart is said to house the mind and serve as the seat of emotions. This point allows us to break through any emotional blocks or bitterness to reestablish order, restoring emotions to their rightful mental state of warmth and peace. This is also an important point for repairing cognition following brain damage due to opioid use, further restoring us to our true self.

HT 7
TCM name: Spirit Gate
Location: On the inside of the wrist, on radial side of the tendon of the flexor carpi ulnaris muscle, on the crease of the wrist.

This is the source acupoint for the Heart. It is a direct gateway to repairing the shen when emotional upset, insomnia, or poor cognition is present.

LU 9
TCM name: Great Abyss
Location: On the crease of the wrist, below the thumb where the radial artery pulsates.

LU 9 is the source point of qi for the Metal element. It is used to establish healthy boundaries broken by abuse. This is an excellent point to stimulate when reestablishing self-dignity and integrity in the aftermath of the lying, stealing, and cheating associated with the abyss of addiction.

CHAPTER 6

Nutrition and Supplements

Rebuilding the Body's Reserves

I t is well established that chronic opioid use leads to severe nutritional deficiencies that can linger in those working to recover.[110] If
left unaddressed, these nutritional deficiencies can make recovery more
difficult and contribute to low energy, low mood, and long-term health
problems.

You can target specific nutritional deficiencies with supplements,
including everything from vitamins and minerals to amino acids, and
we'll talk about some of the most broadly useful ones later in this
chapter. If you are able to identify the patterns that indicate specific
imbalances in your energetic organ systems (see page 29), you can
tailor your diet to correct those imbalances and bring your body back
to a state of equilibrium and health. We'll discuss the patterns that are
most common among opioid users.

You can also adopt healthy eating habits, which, not unsur-
prisingly, go a long way toward rebuilding the body and correcting
imbalances.

RAW FOODS: WESTERN VERSUS TCM PERSPECTIVES

Many well-intentioned health food proponents have touted the benefits of raw foods and the importance of the enzymes found in raw foods for digestion. According to TCM, this logic has three errors:

1. No one dietary guideline is going to be correct for all individuals.

2. Raw foods tend to have cold energy, and overconsumption of them can tax the Spleen and lead to Spleen qi deficiency. In TCM, the Spleen is paired with the Stomach and is central in the proper digestion and absorption of food. With Spleen qi deficiency, digestion and absorption will be poor. Therefore, a raw-foods diet will tend to have the opposite effect on your health than what is desired.

3. People who consume large amounts of raw foods often have loose bowel movements throughout the day, and they see this as a sign that their digestive system is purging more efficiently due to the enzymes found in raw food. In fact, according to TCM, loose bowel movements are a symptom of Spleen damage, not an indicator of healthy enzyme levels.

TCM Food Therapy

There is no lack of information on healthy foods and how to prepare them, so we will not review every bit of that detail. But we are approaching the topic of opioid abuse recovery from the perspective of TCM, which conceptualizes healthy eating in a way that differs from the common Western perspective.

Diet is a vital component of TCM. In fact, nutritional therapy, or food therapy, is one of the five main TCM branches — the others are acupuncture, herbal medicine, tui na (therapeutic massage), and qi gong (energy healing). Foods, just like herbs, have different energetic qualities; they can be warming or cooling, for example, or they can support yin or yang. A TCM practitioner is just as likely to prescribe dietary therapy as she or he is to prescribe herbs or acupuncture.

In terms of Chinese nutritional guidelines, no food is inherently "good" or "bad." Instead, foods are simply appropriate or not appropriate for an individual, depending on each person's unique constitution, energetic balance, and state of health. For example, yang warming tonic foods would be quite beneficial for an individual who is cold and fatigued; however, the same nourishing, warming foods would cause irritation and headaches in someone who is thirsty and experiencing night sweats, as is seen in cases of yin deficiency.

Throughout this book, we've looked at some of the more common imbalances that are seen in cases of extended opioid use. Food therapy can be a valuable partner in correcting these imbalances, and the following pages will show you which kinds of foods are best for these specific imbalances. However, people in the early stages of recovery from opioid dependency often experience lack of appetite and nausea. For them, food therapy may not seem like an attractive option. Keep in mind that lack of appetite and nausea are classic symptoms of Spleen qi deficiency. Once this energetic imbalance is resolved (see page 160 for a targeted protocol), food therapy can be a tremendously valuable tool in rebuilding a person's health, energy, and outlook.

FOOD THERAPY FOR KIDNEY YIN DEFICIENCY

Because the Kidney energetic system is the root of all yin of the body, foods that nourish Kidney yin would be appropriate for yin deficiency originating in any organ system. Heat is a common symptom of yin deficiency, resulting from a lack of yin's cooling, moistening functions, and many yin-nourishing foods are cooling to help balance that heat. Foods that are overly stimulating, like coffee and spices, should be avoided.

FOODS TO SUPPORT KIDNEY YIN			
	amaranth	millet	string beans
	bananas	mung beans	tofu
	barley	quinoa	watermelon
	beets	rice (preferably brown short grain)	wheat germ
	black beans		white mulberry (fruit)
	goji berry	seaweed	
	grapes	spirulina	
	kidney beans		

FOODS TO AVOID	
	alcohol
	coffee
	fats
	red meat
	spices

FOOD THERAPY FOR KIDNEY YANG OR QI DEFICIENCY

Foods that are warming support Kidney yang and qi.

FOODS TO SUPPORT KIDNEY YANG	adzuki beans	coconut	mustard leaf
	basil	cumin	onions
	beef	dates	peaches
	black beans	fennel	raspberries
	black pepper	ginger	rosemary
	butter	garlic	sesame seeds
	cherries	guava	shrimp
	chicken	kale	trout
	chili peppers	lamb	vinegar
	cinnamon	lentils	walnuts
	cloves	molasses	winter squash
	cooked fruit	mussels	
FOODS TO AVOID	asparagus		
	dairy		
	eggplant		
	raw fruits or vegetables		
	wheat		

FOOD THERAPY FOR LIVER QI STAGNATION

Liver qi stagnation is a common phenomenon not only among opioid users but in Western culture generally. When Liver qi is congested, it tends to heat up and Liver yin is consumed.

FOODS TO TONIFY LIVER YIN

artichoke
avocado
beef
beets
cardoon
chicken soup
blackberries
blackstrap molasses
blueberries
dates
eggs
gelatin

dark leafy greens (such as kale, spinach, and collards)
kelp
liver
mulberries
nettles
oysters
pork
red grapes
sesame seeds
spirulina

FOODS TO COOL LIVER HEAT

amaranth
celery
cheese
cucumbers
lettuce
mung beans
mung sprouts
millet
mushrooms
nettles
plums

quinoa
radishes (including daikon)
raw green vegetable juices
rhubarb
rye bread
seaweed
tofu
watercress

FOOD THERAPY FOR HEART BLOOD DEFICIENCY

Heart blood deficiency is common among opioid users, as blood is a yin substance and opioid users often have overall yin deficiency. Heart qi deficiency is another common condition, but the influence of nutrition is less impactful for chronic Heart qi deficiency than it is for other organ imbalances (see page 155 for a treatment protocol for Heart qi deficiency).

FOODS TO SUPPORT HEART BLOOD	adzuki beans	fish
	arugula	lamb
	avocado	legumes
	Brussels sprouts (cooked)	mung beans
	chicory	nuts
	cooked/steamed vegetables (including kale)	
FOODS TO EAT ONLY IN MODERATION	cayenne pepper	
	cherry	
	garlic	
	goji berries	
	hawthorn berry	
	mulberry fruit	
	papaya	
	plum	
	rye	
FOODS TO AVOID	hydrogenated oils	
	processed carbohydrates	
	refined vegetable oils	

FOOD THERAPY FOR SPLEEN QI DEFICIENCY AND INTERNAL DAMPNESS

The Spleen system is damaged by cold foods, raw foods, sugar, and fried foods. According to TCM, once Spleen qi is deficient, the body is unable to absorb nutrients, thus rendering efforts to eat well moot.

FOODS TO SUPPORT SPLEEN QI	adzuki beans	millet
	amaranth	pumpkin
	asparagus	radishes
	carrots (cooked, not raw)	rye
	celery (cooked, not raw)	scallions
	garlic	soybeans (cooked, not raw)
	bitter greens (such as arugula and dandelion, but in moderation, as they are cold)	sunflower seeds
		turnips
		winter squash
	horseradish	yams
	kasha	
FOODS TO AVOID	cucumbers	meat
	dairy	refined carbohydrates
	eggs	sweets
	fried foods	tofu
	fruits and fruit juices	watermelon

FOOD THERAPY FOR LUNG QI DEFICIENCY

The Lungs are often affected by dampness; because dampness is closely associated with the Spleen, nutritional recommendations for the Spleen would be appropriate in cases of chronic phlegm in the lungs. The influence of foods is less impactful for chronic Lung qi deficiency than for Spleen or Kidney yin deficiency, but the recommendations below are helpful.

FOODS TO SUPPORT LUNG QI	almonds carrots (cooked, not raw) chard mushrooms	mustard greens onions rice walnuts
FOODS TO EAT ONLY IN MODERATION	cheese duck grapes pears	radishes tangerines water chestnuts
FOODS TO AVOID	black pepper excessive spicy foods such as hot peppers	garlic ginger

Restorative Chicken Soup

A traditional part of Chinese cuisine, medicinal soups are commonly used to promote longevity, good health, and a strong immune system. This slow-cooked soup is a pleasant way to nourish the body and correct deficiencies created by extended opioid use, especially for someone who has not been eating a consistently healthy diet for a time. The soup is wonderfully restorative and can be enjoyed by the entire family. Those recovering from debility should eat 1 cup of soup two times daily for 3 to 6 weeks.

INGREDIENTS

2 ounces medicinal herb mix (page 133)

2 quarts chicken broth

2 cups chopped cooked chicken

¼ cup chopped scallions

1 tablespoon chopped fresh ginger

Salt and freshly ground black pepper

1 cup cooked brown rice or noodles (optional)

2–4 cups chopped vegetables, such as bok choy, broccoli, carrots, or shiitake mushrooms

Chopped cilantro or scallions, for garnish

PREPARATION

Place the herbs in a large pot and pour the broth over them. Bring the broth to a simmer over medium-high heat; once the soup is simmering, reduce the heat to medium-low and let simmer for 30 minutes. Then add the cooked chicken, scallions, and ginger, and season generously with salt and pepper. Simmer the soup for 2 to 4 hours. Add the vegetables in the last 15 to 30 minutes so that they will be tender but not mushy. When the soup is ready, stir in the cooked rice or noodles, if using. Serve hot, garnished with cilantro and/or scallions, if you like.

Medicinal Herb Mix

This herb mix is a classic addition to medicinal soups used to build strength, fortify the immune system, and restore health generally. The herbs used are mainly qi tonic herbs that can benefit all of the organ systems. Jujube dates are added to support the body's absorption of the other herbs and are a vital qi tonic on their own.

INGREDIENTS

1 part astragalus

1 part codonopsis

1 part goji berries

1 part red jujube dates

PREPARATION

Combine all the herbs and mix well. Store the mixture in a cool, dry spot. When you cook with it, note that the goji berries and red dates are edible, but the astragalus and codonopsis are not; tie them up in a cheesecloth bundle that you can easily remove when the soup is ready to be served.

Nutritional Supplements

Most opioid addicts are significantly nutritionally depleted by the time they enter treatment.[111] Adopting a well-balanced whole-foods diet is crucial for maintaining sobriety, but most people will require additional supplementation during the early months of recovery because their bodies have been starved of nutrients for so long.[112] Additionally, the toxic nature of opioids in and of itself damages the tissues of the body, and extra efforts are required to give the body the resources it needs to repair that damage.

These supplements are readily available online and at health-food markets. However, you should consult with your health-care provider before taking any supplements. When you do take them, stay within the dosages recommended on the product labels.

Magnesium supplementation has been shown to lessen many symptoms related to opioid withdrawal, including anxiety, nervous tension, depression, and muscle spasms. Magnesium supplements also improve sleep patterns.[113] You might consider looking for a magnesium-calcium combined supplement, as the body requires calcium in order to absorb magnesium.

Omega-3 fatty acids can aid those recovering from opioid-induced brain damage by supporting the structural component of neuronal membranes in the brain. Omega-3s have also been shown to be beneficial in the treatment of depression, which is commonly seen in the aftermath of opioid addiction.[114]

Probiotics restore the gut flora, which are often damaged by opioid use, and can be beneficial to those experiencing narcotic bowel disorder (see page 202) following withdrawal.[115]

Vitamin B complex helps combat stress and supports the nervous system. This can be an important supplementation in sustaining opioid recovery, as stressors can trigger relapse. Vitamin B has also been shown to combat depression, a symptom that often appears when opioid use is discontinued.[116]

Vitamin C reduces inflammation, which can be helpful for opioid users struggling with chronic pain. Those who have used opioids for a long time will want to bolster their immune system, and vitamin C is beneficial for this also.[117] One clinical study showed that high doses (15,000 to 20,000 mg) of vitamin C daily lessened withdrawal symptoms.[118] However, such extremely high doses of vitamin C daily can cause digestive upset and should not be maintained for more than a few days. From a TCM perspective, vitamin C is quite cold in nature, and high doses have the potential to damage the Spleen.

Zinc can help improve immune system and brain function.[119] Both are damaged by long-term opioid use, so zinc supplementation would be useful for anyone going through recovery to help bring their body back to health.

Amino Acid Supplements

As we discussed in chapter 1, opioid drugs work by binding with the receptor sites for natural opioids in the brain. Over time, with ongoing overstimulation by opioid drugs, the cell membranes at the receptor sites become damaged and the receptors no longer function properly. These tissues are dependent on proteins for repair.

Amino acids are the building blocks of protein and the foundation for neuroregeneration. A nutritious diet rich in protein sources, such as eggs, meat, cheese, and fish, is crucial for good health in any human being. However, people who have suffered from long-term opioid dependency often require more amino acids for cellular repair than could reasonably be provided by food. For them, supplementation during the first few months of their recovery can be helpful.

While food sources of protein contain a wide range of amino acids, there are a few specific ones that are especially helpful in brain function repair and in mitigating some of the negative factors that make recovery challenging, such as poor sleep, depression, poor digestion, inability to concentrate, and cravings.

As is the case with any nutritional supplements, you should consult with your health-care provider before taking amino acid supplements. When you do take them, stay within the recommended dosages on the product labels.

L-Tryptophan and 5-HTP

L-tryptophan and 5-hydroxytryptophan (5-HTP) are necessary for the manufacture of serotonin, a neurotransmitter and the brain's natural antidepressant. Both are naturally occurring amino acids, and L-tryptophan is converted in the body to 5-HTP, which itself is then converted to serotonin. Enhancing serotonin levels through L-tryptophan supplementation aids in opioid recovery in the following ways:

Mood. The body uses serotonin to transmit messages between nerve cells. It appears to play a key role in maintaining balanced mood. Low serotonin levels have been linked to depression.[120]

Anxiety. Serotonin's role in brain function is important in lessening anxiety and general feelings of unease, which can be debilitating to opioid users during the withdrawal period and can trigger relapse in the following months of recovery.[121]

Digestion. Opioid use often leads to constipation. Serotonin is thought to be active in constricting smooth muscles and thus to play an important role in the function of the large intestines.[122]

Sleep. Long-term opioid use disrupts sleep cycles. As the precursor for melatonin, serotonin helps regulate the body's sleep-wake cycles and internal clock.[123]

Gamma-Aminobutyric Acid (GABA)

Gamma-aminobutyric acid (GABA) is the chief inhibitory neurotransmitter of the central nervous system. GABA supplements have often been touted as useful for treating alcoholism, but they can also play an important role in opioid recovery in the following areas:

Stress and anxiety. People in withdrawal often experience emotional stress and anxiety. GABA may help alleviate some of those symptoms.[124]

Cravings. A recent study suggests that GABA may boost impulse control, and thus it may help prevent relapse.[125]

Fatigue. Opioid users in recovery often experience fatigue that can last many months. One study suggests that GABA may help reduce both psychological and physical fatigue.[126]

Muscle spasms. Those detoxing from opioids can experience very uncomfortable muscle spasms. GABA plays an important role in the regulation of muscle tone and can help prevent or ameliorate spasms.[127]

L–Tyrosine

The body uses L-tyrosine to manufacture dopamine, which in turn is used in the manufacture of norepinephrine and epinephrine.[128] Dopamine is our "focus" neurotransmitter; it regulates cognition and is involved with the executive brain functions that help us control impulses and withstand cravings.[129] It also regulates emotion, motivation, and feelings of pleasure.

L-tyrosine, which is essential for the production of dopamine, can be helpful to the recovering opioid user in a couple of ways:

Cravings. Prolonged opioid use causes structural changes in the brain that influence behaviors associated with the massive opioid-induced dopamine release.[130] The importance of cultivating proper dopamine reactions is most apparent when a person in recovery is exposed to stimuli they associate with the opioid use, such as certain people, places, and situations, as the association networks that have evolved in the brain will strongly interlink these environmental cues with opioid use and can prompt a relapse. [131]

Cognition. Extended opioid consumption causes debilitating stress for the brain, negatively affecting cognition. And people in recovery often experience prolonged insomnia, which also can negatively affect cognition. L-tyrosine has been shown to improve cognitive function.[132]

Note: L-tyrosine is contraindicated in those who suffer from melanoma, Grave's disease, phenylketonuria (PKU), chronic migraines, Hashimoto's thyroiditis, high blood pressure, or bipolar disorder.

DL-Phenylalanine

The body uses DL-phenylalanine (DLPA) to convert L-tyrosine to dopamine, and the two are often packaged together in supplement form. DLPA is also key in the synthesis of endorphins, which are the brain's natural, or endogenous, painkillers (see page 15).[133] Therefore, DLPA can be important in combating both dopamine and endorphin deficits — both of which are common in people recovering from opioid dependency.

Note: D- or DL-phenylalanine is contraindicated in those who suffer from melanoma, Grave's disease, phenylketonuria (PKU), chronic migraines, Hashimoto's thyroiditis, high blood pressure, or manic depression (bipolar disorder).

L-Glutamine

L-glutamine is another amino acid that impacts neurotransmission and participates in a variety of metabolic pathways, and it has been the subject of many recent studies. It is a precursor to GABA, and the two are often used together. Here are some of the ways it may be able to aid in opioid addiction recovery:

Digestion. Many of those using opioids experience digestive imbalances that last long after opioid use has stopped. Glutamine has been shown to improve gastrointestinal health by activating the repair of the intestinal lining and protecting it from deterioration. It promotes healthy bowel movements, lessens episodes of diarrhea and irritable bowel syndrome (IBS), and helps heal ulcers.[134]

Memory. Glutamine is essential for nourishing the neuronal synapses responsible for transmitting information in the brain. It can stimulate repair of the damage done to opioid receptors while improving memory, focus, and concentration overall.[135]

Detoxification. Glutamine improves liver and kidney metabolism of cellular toxins resulting from opioid use.[136]

Note: Use caution when taking L-glutamine if you have bipolar disorder, as it can stimulate a manic episode.

PART 2

Protocols
for
TREATMENT

CHAPTER 7

Basic Protocols
Treating Addiction by Correcting Elemental Imbalances

According to TCM, we all embody the characteristics of all five elements — Water, Wood, Fire, Earth, Metal — but most of us have a dominant element, as indicated by our dominant character traits. We display the negative emotional attributes of that element when it is out of balance; conversely, we embody the positive characteristics and personal strengths of that element when we are well and our body and mind are in balance.

Opioid abuse has a strong negative impact on our elemental balance. Elemental imbalances manifest in different ways, depending on the individual. In this chapter, we'll discuss some of the more common manifestations in people suffering from opioid dependency, and we'll look at protocols for treating those imbalances. Recognizing elemental imbalances allows us to craft an effective strategy for addressing the emotional disorders that contribute to continuing opioid dependency, so that we can overcome our addiction and regain balance and wellness. These strategies can include acupuncture, acupressure, herbs, essential oils, nutrition, exercise, meditation, and more.

Let's take a look.

WORK WITH A PROFESSIONAL

Some of the therapies discussed in these protocols can be self-administered, such as herbs, acupressure, and flower essences. Others must be administered by a professional, such as a licensed acupuncturist. Ultimately, the responsibility for a full recovery from opioid use/abuse lies in the hands of the patient. No practitioner from any medicinal tradition can "fix" you, and no single remedy is a complete cure for addiction. The protocols detailed in these pages are intended to empower patients so that they can more clearly understand their treatment options and engage in their own healing. They are not "stand-alone" treatments; anyone looking to overcome opioid dependency should work with local health-care guidance to develop a plan of action for recovery.

Water/Kidney Imbalances

Water element imbalances are common in opioid dependency because stress consumes Kidney yin, and most opioid use is predicated on some type of stress, whether physical, social, or psychological. Ongoing opioid use and withdrawal are also stressful, exacerbating any yin deficiency. The Kidneys and the Water element are linked, so Water imbalances and Kidney deficiencies go hand in hand. Some practitioners would call this type of Kidney deficiency adrenal fatigue, and indeed, studies have shown that chronic opioid use results in adrenal insufficiencies.[137]

From a TCM perspective, when opioids contribute to Kidney deficiency and a Water element imbalance, anxiety and panic attacks result. From a Western perspective, prolonged use of opioids damages neurotransmitters in the brain that play a central role in the anxiety response, which has the same effect.[138] In either case, using opioids nullifies anxiety, but once they are discontinued, feelings of unease, anxiety, and eventually panic begin to surface. These feelings contribute to cravings for opioids and increase the chance of relapse.[139]

Because the Water element governs willpower, and giving up an opioid dependency requires tremendous willpower, reinforcing the Kidney energetic system becomes especially important during withdrawal and recovery (see page 171). It's also important to address adrenal fatigue (see page 201).

The strengths of individuals who embody Water element attributes are resilience and the ability to overcome inevitable obstacles of recovery. Like the waters of a lake, their thoughts run deep and they bestow calm energy and deep wisdom on those who are in their company. Upon recovery of health and balance, the person's clear insight and deep perception, which have been fortified by the experiences he or she has gained through dependency and recovery, lead to a purpose-filled life.

Kidney Yin Deficiency

The yin of the body originates with Kidney yin; therefore, a yin deficiency developing in any organ system in the body will indicate Kidney yin deficiency.

PATTERNS OF KIDNEY YIN DEFICIENCY

- Afternoon or evening sweats
- Dry mouth or throat
- Thirst
- Feeling of fever in afternoon or evening
- Tinnitus (constant ringing in ears)
- Pain or dull ache in the lower back
- Aching bones
- Weakness in the knees or lower back

Self-Treatment Options for Kidney Yin Deficiency

CLINIC FORMULA: Opioid Yin Tonic

PATENT FORMULA: *liu wei huang wan*

ACUPRESSURE POINT: KI 3 (page 62)

SINGLE HERBS: fo-ti (page 85), goji (page 86), privet fruit (page 91), schisandra (page 93)

ESSENTIAL OILS: any of those correlating to the Water element with a cooling nature, such as geranium (page 108), lavender (page 110), or marjoram (page 112)

OPIOID YIN TONIC

This formula contains nourishing yin tonic herbs along with herbs that address common aspects of yin deficiency seen in addiction recovery, such as sweating and thirst. It would be appropriate for those who are experiencing Kidney yin deficiency symptoms and would be used over a matter of many months until the symptoms subside. This formula is cooling and nourishing for blood and organ tissue but is not cold in nature. For dosages, follow the recommendation of your licensed practitioner.

CHINESE NAME	ENGLISH NAME	PERCENTAGE OF FORMULA
Shu di huang	Rehmannia (cooked)	14.9%
Shan zhu yu	Cornus	8.9%
Shan yao	Dioscorea	8.6%
Sang ye	Mulberry leaf	8.3%
Nu zhen zi	Ligustrum	8.0%
Mu dan pi (su)	Moutan	6.5%
Fu ling	Poria	6.2%
Ze xie	Alisma	5.9%
He shou wu	Fo-ti	5.6%
Ge gen (fen ge gen)	Pueraria root	5.3%
Gou qi zi	Lycium fruit	5.0%
Gu sui bu	Drynaria	4.7%
Yin chai hu	Stellaria root	4.4%
Ju hua	Chrysanthemum	4.1%
Long yan rou	Longan fruit	3.6%

Kidney Yang Deficiency

The Kidneys are also the origination point of yang in the body, and yang deficiency anywhere in the body can originate from Kidney yang. Yin is the material basis of yang, so a yin deficiency sometimes leads to a yang deficiency, and a yang deficiency is always indicative of a yin deficiency. Yang deficiency patterns present with slowed metabolic processes, such as hypothyroidism or even shallow breath. Kidney yang deficiency affects many aspects of health, including core energy, sexual energy, lower back strength, knee strength, hair health, and reproductive health. Many people who are kidney deficient experience a drop in energy in the afternoon around 3:00 p.m.

Someone suffering from a yang deficiency may look pale or anemic, may have dark circles under his eyes, and will have a weak voice. Women who are yang deficient will likely have pale or watery menstrual blood and backaches associated with their period.

PATTERNS OF KIDNEY YANG DEFICIENCY

- Pain or dull ache in the lower back
- Soreness in the knees
- Weakness in the lower limbs
- Coldness of the body, especially the hands and feet
- Social withdrawal
- A tendency to catch colds easily
- Impotence
- Infertility
- Loose morning stools
- Frequent urination
- Edema
- Anxiety, panic attacks, and fearfulness

Self-Treatment Options for Kidney Yang Deficiency

CLINIC FORMULA: Opioid Yang Tonic

PATENT FORMULA: *you gui wan*

ACUPRESSURE POINTS: KI 3, KI 6 (page 62)

SINGLE HERBS: fo-ti (page 85), privet fruit (page 91), reishi (page 92)

ESSENTIAL OILS: any of those correlating to the Water element with a warming nature, such as basil (page 102), cinnamon leaf (page 103), or nutmeg (page 113)

Follow the suggestions for treating adrenal exhaustion (page 201)

OPIOID YANG TONIC

This formula contains warming yang tonic herbs along with herbs that address common aspects of yang deficiency seen in addiction recovery, such as adrenal fatigue. It would be used in cases of where the patient feels chronically cold. If heat symptoms of yin deficiency are present, such as sweating and thirst, one would combine the yin and yang formulas and take each at half strength so not to exacerbate the yin deficiency. For dosages, follow the recommendation of your licensed practitioner.

CHINESE NAME	ENGLISH NAME	PERCENTAGE OF FORMULA
Shu di huang	Rehmannia (cooked)	14.3%
Tu si zi	Cuscuta seed	14%
Shan yao	Dioscorea	8.3%
Yin yang huo	Epimedium	7.4%
Ze xie	Alisma	7.1%
Gou qi zi	Lycium fruit	6.9%
Wu wei zi	Schisandra	6.6%
Shan zhu yu	Cornus	6.3%
Mu dan pi (su)	Moutan	6.0%
Gui zhi	Cinnamon twigs	5.7%
Bu gu zhi	Psoralea	5.4%
Fu ling	Poria	4.6%
Du zhong	Eucommia	4.0%
Huang jing (jiu)	Polygonatum (Solomon's seal)	3.4%

Water Element Imbalance

PATIENT: Linda S., female, 32 years old

Linda, a pharmaceutical sales representative who described herself as having a Type A personality, arrived at my office after almost 2 years of opioid use following a skiing accident that injured her lower back. While her back pain had dissipated greatly, her cravings for opioids had only grown. Linda's story was a common one: she was able to continue her opioid use by doctor shopping. When one prescription ran out, she would simply visit another doctor complaining about severe pain to gain another prescription. Linda explained how she had gone from being a confident and successful young woman to an unmotivated individual experiencing anxiety and panic attacks on a regular basis.

Luckily, her family lived close by and noticed changes in Linda's personality. After 6 months of suspicions, they pieced together their conclusion of ongoing drug use. The family organized an intervention, during which their powerful group admonition helped Linda recognize the truth of the matter. In the weeks that followed, she tried to quit cold turkey several times, but her efforts resulted in severe nausea, sweating, terror, and an eventual return to the seductive narcotic.

After checking her pulse at several points and examining her tongue, I determined that Linda had Kidney yin deficiency. The Kidney organ system belongs to the Water element. When the Water element is out of balance, the associated emotion is fear, as seen with Linda's chronic anxiety and panic attacks. Linda also reported that, about 6 months earlier, she had begun waking with night terrors, covered in sweat. Those with Kidney yin deficiency experience worsened symptoms at night. Her left medial pulse was tight and pounding, suggesting Liver heat. The tip of her tongue was bright red, indicating Heart heat, and it is common in cases of insomnia for Liver heat to rise and attack the Heart.

A diagnosis of a Liver imbalance was also supported by the fact that Linda reportedly went from being an ambitious young woman with goals and dreams to being an unmotivated individual with little hope or vision for the future. The liver is involved with opioid metabolism, and chronic use of them often results in Liver qi stagnation and Liver yin deficiency. The Kidney organ system is the basis of all yin in the body, and Liver yin deficiency was indicated by the peeling yellow areas on the side of Linda's tongue.

Linda's case demonstrates how all of the organ systems are interconnected and must be brought in to harmony. Even Linda's initial injury played in to her diagnosis: an individual with Kidney deficiency would have a weak back.

With these findings, Linda and I set forth in creating a treatment strategy that would fit into her life.

The Treatment Protocol
WEEKS 1 AND 2

- ACUPUNCTURE: three times per week
- CLINIC FORMULAS FOR WITHDRAWAL: Quell Quease (page 175), Calm Mind (page 176), and Ease Detox (page 177)

WEEKS 3 TO 8

- ACUPUNCTURE: two times per week
- CLINIC FORMULAS: Opioid Liver Balancer (page 150), Opioid Yin Tonic (page 143), and Opioid Brain Tonic (page 198)
- SUPPLEMENTS: amino acid blend of L-tryptophan and 5-HTP, L-tyrosine, and DL-phenylalanine (DLPA) at the recommended doses listed on the product label for 6 weeks

ONGOING SELF-TREATMENT

- ACUPRESSURE: two or three times per day on points KI 3 (page 62), HT 7 and HT 8 (page 64), PER 7 and PER 8 (page 64), LV 2 and LV 3 (page 63), and ST 36 (page 65)
- ESSENTIAL OILS: any of those correlating to the Water element with a cooling nature, such as geranium (page 108), lavender (page 110), or marjoram (page 112)
- MEDITATION: Five Element Meditation (page 28) twice per day

Linda was fortunate enough to have accrued vacation days from her job. She was also fortunate in having an M.D. who helped her set a schedule for weaning off the opioids over the first 8 weeks of recovery. She decided to take the first week of treatment off from work and was able to come for an acupuncture treatment three times. Her withdrawal symptoms were minimal, but she was still experiencing her original symptoms of anxiety and insomnia, which did not begin to ease up until week 8. Thereafter, she continued the herbal therapy and received acupuncture one time per week for 6 more months, at which point she was free of drug cravings, anxiety, and sleep problems. Linda continued to visit the acupuncture clinic one or two times per month for 2 more years, during which time she received herbal prescriptions based on her presentation of imbalances. She was eventually restored to her original enthusiastic, energetic self.

Wood/Liver Imbalances

The organ system associated with the Wood element is the Liver. Because opioids are broken down in the liver, most people who take opioids for an extended period experience some level of liver damage. Damage to the liver causes a person to begin to harbor the negative feelings of the Wood element: anger, frustration, and resentment. Liver qi stagnation often results.

People who are prone to Wood imbalances tend to be more impulsive and reckless than most; this can create a predisposition to drug use. During withdrawal and early recovery, a Wood persona with Liver qi stagnation will be aggressive, confrontational, and angry at the world. Additionally, such people often display a false sense of confidence and arrogance that blocks them from being able to accept advice and wise teachings from others; this impedes recovery efforts.

As recovery progresses, those of the Wood type will begin to show their true nature as confident and highly motivated. Like a tree, they will develop attributes of flexibility and adaptability when the disruptive winds of life blow. They tend to have great foresight, and their ability to envision the future will allow them to create a strategic plan for a brighter future. As the Liver is soothed, their aggression turns to motivation, healthy competitiveness, and productive ambition. Once the post-withdrawal exhaustion lifts, those with the Wood personality type can burst forward with assertive drive and implement positive change in their life.

Liver Qi Stagnation

The Liver system is very powerful according to TCM; it is a yin organ, but it can be quite yang and reactive when it's not happy and soothed. The Liver controls the smooth flow of qi throughout the body, which is crucial to the health of all of the organ systems. Left unchecked, Liver qi stagnation and imbalance will develop into aggression that is unleashed on other organ systems. Liver qi stagnation is arguably the most common pattern of imbalance in Western culture.

SYMPTOMS OF LIVER QI STAGNATION

- Anger, irritability, and frustration
- Feeling stuck emotionally
- Depression
- Anxiety, stress
- Tenderness around the ribs
- Hard-to-swallow lump in throat
- Sighing often

Self-Treatment Options for Liver Qi Stagnation

CLINIC FORMULA: Opioid Liver Balancer (page 150)

PATENT FORMULA: *xiao yao wan*

ACUPRESSURE POINTS: LV 2 and LV 3 (page 63), LI 4 (page 66)

SINGLE HERBS: dandelion (page 83), fo-ti (page 85), schisandra (page 93), white peony (page 95), yellow dock (page 97)

ESSENTIAL OILS: any of those correlating to the Wood element, including fennel (page 107), marjoram (page 112), or Mandarin Orange/Tangerine (page 111)

Follow the suggestions for detoxification (page 178)

CLINIC FORMULA: OPIOID LIVER BALANCER

This formula nourishes and soothes the Liver while helping to calm the mind. It restores the Liver's function of eliminating toxins. It would be most appropriate for people displaying indications of Liver qi stagnation, such as being quick to anger and frustration. It would be used over many months until symptoms have been resolved. For dosages, follow the recommendation of your licensed practitioner.

CHINESE NAME	ENGLISH NAME	PERCENTAGE OF FORMULA
Xuan shen	Scrophularia	13.6%
Chai hu	Bupleurum	11.2%
Bai shao	White peony	10.8%
Xia ku cao	Spica prunellae	10.5%
Tian hua fen	Trichosanthes root	10.2%
Bai ji li	Tribulus	9.8%
Zhi mu	Anemarrhena rhizome	7.8%
Xiang fu	Cyperus rhizome	6.4%
He shou wu (zhi)	Fo-ti	4.4%
Han lian cao	Eclipta	4.1%
Qing pi	Citrus peel (green)	3.4%
Pu gong ying	Dandelion	2.7%
Xiao hui xiang	Fennel fruit	2.0%
Chen pi (ju pi)	Citrus peel (mature)	1.4%
Dang gui (shen)	Dong gui	1.0%
Suan zao ren	Zizyphus	0.7%

Wood Element Imbalance

PATIENT: Walter V., male, 58 years old

Standing over 6 feet tall with a muscular build, Walter entered my office in a huff; he was frustrated by the lengthy patient questionnaire that he was required to fill out as a new patient. He made his complaint quite clear in a booming voice. For a moment I was put back on my heels, but I regained my composure as I recognized the Wood element personality. I pivoted from feeling attacked to feeling thankful for the diagnostic clues that would help me form an effective treatment plan for this patient.

As Walter began to share his story, more clues began to emerge. Though he had calmed down, his normal speaking voice sounded like a shout; his face was drooping on one side, likely due to a palsy resulting from a stroke; and the knuckles on his left hand were slightly deformed from arthritis. Before he had finished his first sentence, I had formed a large part of his diagnosis as long-standing Liver qi stagnation.

As it turned out, Walter had suffered a stroke 1 year earlier and had largely recovered with intensive physical therapy and medication. He had fallen during the stroke and fractured his arm, leading to an opioid prescription. A year later the pain was long gone, but he had become psychologically dependent on the drugs. He was angry at the doctor who prescribed the opioids, at his estranged wife for leaving him following the stroke, and at God for bestowing these curses upon him.

It was important that I clearly explain to Walter that his predicament was due to chronic illness. He had come to me expecting a speedy and painless opioid withdrawal. A deeper understanding of his condition would allow him to choose a short course of treatment for withdrawal only, or a longer course of treatment wherein he could achieve true, long-standing wellness.

His new-patient intake had indicated that Walter had been diagnosed 8 years earlier with high blood pressure and was taking a blood-thinning medication. Because 1 in 3 adults in the United States has high blood pressure,[140] patients often do not perceive of it as a significant health issue. Walter was aware that 80 percent of stroke victims had previously been diagnosed with high blood pressure,[141] but he did not link that diagnosis with his stroke since his blood pressure had been controlled with medication. I explained that it had first taken years of Liver imbalance for high blood pressure to develop in the first case. Additionally, I shared that in TCM a stroke is called a Wind-Stroke and is considered to result from internal wind created by Liver heat; his stroke, I told him, was due to a chronic condition that had been unchecked for over a decade, not a random bolt of lightning sent by God to strike him down.

A full evaluation of Walter's tongue and pulse, along with his health history, painted a rather complicated picture of Liver qi stagnation, Kidney and Liver yin deficiency, and Heart heat. The opioid withdrawal process would take only about 3 or 4 weeks, but addressing his chronic health imbalances would take many months of acupuncture and herbal therapy. It was a great deal of information for Walter to digest, and we decided to begin with his opioid detoxification regimen while saving discussion of his long-term health issues for later.

Determined to rid himself of his addiction quickly, Walter wanted to quit the pain meds cold turkey that very day. I urged him to wean off the medications over at least 1 week's time. (Unfortunately, because he had begun to purchase his opioids illegally several months prior when his prescriptions ran out, Walter did not have a prescribing physician to aid him with the weaning process.) He conceded, and we began our work together.

The Treatment Protocol
WEEKS 1 AND 2
- ACUPUNCTURE: three or four times per week
- CLINIC FORMULAS FOR WITHDRAWAL: Quell Quease (page 175), Calm Mind (page 176), and Ease Detox (page 177)

WEEKS 3 AND 4

- ACUPUNCTURE: two times per week
- CLINIC FORMULA: Opioid Liver Balancer (page 150)
- SUPPLEMENTS: amino acid blend of L-tryptophan and 5-HTP, L-tyrosine, and DL-phenylalanine (DLPA) at the recommended doses listed on the product label for 6 weeks

MONTHS 2 TO 5

- ACUPUNCTURE: once or twice per week
- CLINIC FORMULA: Opioid Liver Balancer (page 150)
- SINGLE HERBS: hawthorn (page 86) and motherwort (page 89)

It would have been beneficial for Walter to practice self-treatment options such as meditation and acupressure, but they were not appealing to him. I was keen on him using my Heart Tonic herb formula, as it contained beneficial blood-moving Chinese herbs, but this caused the doctor who prescribed his blood-thinning medication concern. Also, Walter protested at the prospect of making and drinking teas; therefore, we decided on just the hawthorn leaf and flower capsules and the motherwort capsules.

To his credit, Walter attended his acupuncture sessions regularly and took his herb capsules consistently. His pulse lost its tight, wiry quality, and he reported that he felt much less stressed and frustrated with life in general. He was especially pleased that we were able to completely resolve the bit of paralysis that had remained in his face. His doctor was able to lower his dosage of blood pressure medication, but we were not able to reverse the damage already done. Similarly, we were able to alleviate the arthritic pain in his fingers, but the physical deformity remained. All in all, we were satisfied with the outcome. Walter continued to visit my community acupuncture clinic every few weeks for several more years, during which time he was able to maintain his sobriety and health improvements without regression.

Fire/Heart Imbalances

The yin organ associated with the Fire element is the Heart, which is said to house the mind and is associated with all emotions. Those who have a tendency toward Fire element imbalances can be especially prone to addiction because they tend to crave mind-altering substances and love to be the life of a party. Joy is the emotion associated with the Fire element, but in its negative aspect, joy becomes mania. During the early stages of dependency, opioids are known to induce a sense of euphoria akin to mania. Prolonged euphoria will damage the Heart system and create an imbalance of the Fire element.

The Fire element is unique in correlating to a conceptual organ system called San Jiao (Triple Burner). The San Jiao is partly responsible for moderating our body temperature on a physical level. Emotionally, a Fire element imbalance affecting the San Jiao can cause people to have emotions that fluctuate vastly; they can be warm and endearing one moment, cold and distant the next.

While the poetic association between love and the heart is well-known all over the world, love in TCM is directly related to the Heart: heartbreak can lead to Heart damage. The Fire element also encompasses the Pericardium (the membrane that encloses the heart), which is referred to as the "heart protector." The Heart is unique as the only organ in the body that has an organ assigned for its protection. The Pericardium acts as a shield, absorbing personal emotional attacks. It also acts as a gate that opens (to allow for love to flow to the Heart) and closes (to protect the Heart from insult). If it is stuck open, an individual is especially vulnerable to emotional attacks. If it is stuck closed, an individual is unable to accept love.

As someone with dominant Fire-type personality traits begins to recover from dependency, he or she begins to reclaim joy. Easy conversation, a propensity for emotional warmth, and natural magnetism will allow this person to build a strong network of friends and family who support the recovery effort. This type of recovering addict will also tend to have a great sense of humor and enthusiasm. The Fire element, associated with summer, reflects warmth and abundance. Summer is when crops ripen and are harvested, and the Fire persona holds great potential for a life in which goals, hopes, and dreams come to full fruition.

Heart Blood and Qi Deficiency

The energetic organ system referred to as the Heart in Chinese medicine is quite similar to the western idea of the physical heart, but it also contributes greatly to emotional stability. In order to function properly, the Heart must receive abundant qi and blood so that it is nourished.

Self-Treatment Options for Heart Blood and Qi Deficiency

CLINIC FORMULA: Opioid Heart Tonic (page 156)

PATENT FORMULA: *tianwang buxin dan*

ACUPRESSURE POINTS: HT 7 and HT 8 (page 64), PER 6 and PER 7 (page 64)

SINGLE HERBS: hawthorn (page 86), motherwort (page 89), red sage (page 92), schisandra (page 93)

ESSENTIAL OILS: any of those correlating to the Fire element, including cinnamon leaf (page 103), clary sage (page 104), or frankincense (page 107)

OPIOID HEART TONIC

This tonic formula specifically repairs damage to the heart muscle and related tissues due to chronic opioid misuse or overdose. In addition to nourishing the heart, it moves blood and resolves blood stagnation. It also helps to clear heart heat, which is commonly seen in conjunction with sleep disturbances in people recovering from opioid abuse. The formula would be taken for 6 to 8 months, or until the symptoms resolve. For dosages, follow the recommendation of your licensed practitioner.

CHINESE NAME	ENGLISH NAME	PERCENTAGE OF FORMULA
Ren shen (hong)	Ginseng	11.3%
He shou wu	Fo-ti	10.8%
Wu wei zi	Schisandra	10.3%
Bai zi ren	Biota seed	9.8%
Shan zha	Crataegus	9.8%
Sheng di huang	Rehmannia (fresh)	9.8%
Dang gui (shen)	Dong gui	9.3%
Dan shen	Salvia root	8.8%
Yuan zhi	Polygala	8.3%
Fu shen	Poria	6.4%
Da zao (hong)	Jujube dates (red)	2.9%
Suan zao ren	Zizyphus	2.5%

Fire Element Imbalance
PATIENT: Janis R., female, 52 years old

Janis, a 52-year-old female, was referred to me after she had been in an automobile accident in which she sustained a back injury and was subsequently prescribed opioids. It had been 6 weeks since the incident, and the prescribing physician would write only one more script for her, allowing her the opportunity to wean off the medication. The problem was that she was still in pain and felt that she had become emotionally dependent on the narcotics. The healing strategy was obvious: alleviate pain and balance the emotions.

The pain aspect of the treatment process was straightforward. I prescribed Janis my clinic pain formula, which contains anti-inflammatory herbs such as turmeric, along with herbs that move blood and qi, as pain cannot manifest in the body without stagnation of blood and/or qi. Her pain was in her lower back located along the Bladder channel and the Du (Governing) channel (which runs over the spinal cord and brain), so I chose acupuncture points along those channels, along with other points that increase circulation. I also instructed her to apply a topical spray infused with healing herbs and essential oils to guide the remedies to the channels of the back.

The emotional balancing would prove to be more complicated. During the initial patient intake, Janis alternated from expressing warm feelings toward her children and grandchildren to explosive outbursts related to her accident and her suffering. Her hot-and-cold emotions continued during the initial weeks of treatment: she would sometimes express gratitude for the healing assistance, and other times strike out over the lack of quick progress. Along with physical symptoms such as palpitations, insomnia, and a burning tongue, it was clear that we would need to pay close attention to the Fire element to reach the best outcomes. In TCM, the Heart houses the mind during sleep. Unlike other elements, the Heart plays a role in all emotional imbalances. I instructed Janis to apply a carefully chosen mix of essential oils to specific acupoints to bring balance to the Heart.

While the Fire element has a propensity for flaring up when out of balance, so too does the Liver organ of the Wood element. Stress, toxins, and anger can lead to Liver qi stagnation. Beyond anger and frustration, Janis had been struggling with irregular bleeding and mood swings, which she associated with menopause. According to the ancient theories of TCM, the Liver controls the menstrual blood. In addition to Janis's outward symptoms, her left middle pulse was tight and hard when palpated, further indicating Liver congestion. It is widely understood that opioids can have a negative impact on the liver, but the damage often occurs because many opioids are combined with the popular analgesic acetaminophen (which in large doses can be toxic to the liver).[142]

The Treatment Protocol

WEEKS 1 TO 3
- ACUPUNCTURE: three times per week
- CLINIC FORMULAS FOR WITHDRAWAL: Quell Quease (page 175), Calm Mind (page 176), and Ease Detox (page 177)

WEEKS 4 TO 11
- ACUPUNCTURE: two times per week
- CLINIC FORMULAS: Opioid Liver Balancer (page 150) and Opioid Brain Tonic (page 198)
- SUPPLEMENTS: amino acid blend of L-tryptophan and 5-HTP, L-tyrosine, and DL-phenylalanine (DLPA) at the recommended doses listed on the product label for 6 weeks

ONGOING SELF-TREATMENT
- ACUPRESSURE: two or three times per day on points HT 7 and HT 8 (page 64), PER 7 and PER 8 (page 64), LV 2 and LV 3 (page 63), and ST 36 (page 65)
- ESSENTIAL OILS: any of those correlating to the Fire element (page 100)
- MEDITATION: Five Element Meditation (page 28) twice per day

Janis came in for treatment three times per week for the first 3 weeks, and then cut down to two times per week for an additional 8 weeks. During weeks 1 through 3 she took formulas containing calming herbs as she weaned off of her opioid medication. While at this stage I considered adding an adaptogen formula, Janis's emotions were leveling off quite nicely and we decided to reserve it for later, and only if needed, since she was already taking three formulas. At the end of the 11-week course of treatment, Janis had remained pain-free for over 2 weeks. I instructed her to continue the herbs for another 3 months and to come in for a treatment one time per month. At this stage I often release patients with instruction to simply schedule an appointment if they need to; however, I am much more guarded with patients coming off opioids and like to make certain that they are staying the course. Janis had a great outcome due to her commitment to wellness and excellent patient compliance.

Earth/Spleen Imbalances

The emotion related to the Earth element is worry. Earth-type opioid addicts will be fraught with fretful notions that they will be unable to stop ruminating about. While worrying does nothing to change a situation, their obsessive contemplations will keep them up at night and consume them during the day. This type of dominant personality is susceptible to developing obsessive-compulsive disorder (OCD). Studies suggest that people with OCD have a greater risk of developing substance abuse, as the ritualistic nature of substance use can appeal to those with OCD.[143]

Those with an Earth-dominant personality will often complain that they do not feel grounded to the earth, and they will appear to be disorganized. With addiction, this persona may seem fretful to the point of being meddlesome or clingy.

Luckily, attributes associated with the Earth element can work to a person's advantage after detoxing from opioids. Earth types are naturally very popular, nurturing, and empathetic; they are great listeners and can rebuild social networks and family ties easily following recovery. Instead of meddling or worrying, they develop innate abilities as natural facilitators who bring people together. Additionally, learning and intellect are attributed to Earth energies; this persona can quickly learn new and positive lifestyle patterns, adapting to a sober life easily.

Spleen Qi Deficiency

The pattern of Spleen qi deficiency is central to all other Spleen disharmonies; in fact, it is the precursor to all Spleen imbalances. If Spleen qi deficiency is not properly treated, it can lead to more serious patterns of imbalance. Any Spleen imbalance therefore indicates some form of Spleen qi deficiency.

Self-Treatment Options for Spleen Qi Deficiency

CLINIC FORMULA: Opioid Spleen Tonic (page 161)

PATENT FORMULA: *gui pi tang*

ACUPRESSURE POINTS: SP 3, SP 6, and SP 9 (page 65); ST 36 (page 65)

SINGLE HERBS: astragalus (page 80), codonopsis (page 83), elecampane (page 84)

ESSENTIAL OILS: any of those correlating to the Earth element, including anise seed (page 101), coriander (page 105), or fennel (page 107)

Follow the suggestions for addressing poor digestion (page 202) and fatigue (page 199)

OPIOID SPLEEN TONIC

This herbal formula contains nourishing Spleen tonic herbs that reinforce qi. Because it addresses an organ-level imbalance, it would take several months of use to resolve the deficiency/imbalance. This formula is also appropriate for treating internal dampness, as the Spleen is implicit in this condition. For dosages, follow the recommendation of your licensed practitioner.

CHINESE NAME	ENGLISH NAME	PERCENTAGE OF FORMULA
Dang shen	Codonopsis	14%
Huang qi (bei)	Astragalus root	12.7%
Shan yao	Dioscorea	12.7%
Bai zhu	Atractylodes (alba)	12.1%
Shan zha	Crataegus	9.2%
Yi yi ren	Coix	8.7%
Da zao (hong)	Jujube dates (red)	6.9%
Cang zhu	Atractylodes	6.4%
Chen pi (ju pi)	Citrus peel (mature)	4.6%
Xiang fu	Cyperus rhizome	4.0%
Pei lan	Eupatorium	3.5%
Fu ling	Poria	2.9%
Huo xiang	Agastache	2.3%

Earth Element Imbalance

PATIENT: Sarah C., female, 20 years old

Accompanied by her mother, Sarah appeared shy, thin, and frail as she entered the office. She sat quietly, looking away as her mother explained her predicament: Sarah had struggled with anorexia through-out high school and developed an opioid dependence during her first year of college, procuring the drugs from illicit sources around campus. When I inquired about her childhood, Sarah's mother revealed that Sarah was born prematurely. Her mother nearly cried as she explained that it was necessary to leave Sarah in the neonatal unit for 2 months, making breastfeeding impossible. Sarah listened pensively as she gently pulled her fingers down through her hair, wadded strands into small balls, and placed them on her lap.

I turned my focus to Sarah and addressed her directly, asking for details. She answered only after her mother took her hand and began to reassure her in a melodic voice usually reserved for addressing babies. After a bit of stroking and cooing, Sarah began to open up. She described the tormenting feelings of ongoing anxiety that she experienced when her college roommate would not keep the room organized the way she liked. This caused her to fret throughout the night and lose sleep. The semester break was fraught with fights with her mother, who discovered that her reliably A student was barely making C's. Sarah begged her mother to allow her to return home and attend a local college, to no avail. The opioid use began shortly after she returned to campus. She failed most of her second-semester classes, and it was agreed that she should return home.

For the Earth element to develop correctly, a baby must be nour-ished and nurtured, especially in utero and during the newborn phase. A baby's bond with her mother, or lack thereof, plays an especially important role in her ability to feel safe and grow to become an inde-pendent and productive adult. The Spleen organ system is the yin organ of the Earth element and is responsible for the metabolism and absorption of food. The early events of Sarah's life, including the fact that she was born before her Earth element was fully formed, created a predisposition to an Earth-element personality disorder. The emotion linked to the Earth element is worry, and those lacking in Earth can develop OCD.

Sarah's eating and attachment disorders were further symptoms forming this diagnosis; however, I was especially concerned by the mother's doting over her adult daughter. Overmothering is just as detrimental as undermothering when it comes to the health of a child's Earth element. This was obviously a long-standing contributor to the disorder, but not something that I could address in my position. I had long known the TCM saying "When treating children, first treat the mother." In our culture, many would see this as an attempt to blame the mother for a child's behavior. As a mother myself, however, I know that mothers tend to be self-sacrificing and put the needs of their children in front of their own. Therefore, I understand that a mother who is not supported well cannot care for her children to her highest capacity.

The Treatment Protocol

MONTH 1

- ACUPUNCTURE: three times per week
- CLINIC FORMULAS FOR WITHDRAWAL: Quell Quease (page 175), Calm Mind (page 176), and Ease Detox (page 177)
- OTHER CLINIC FORMULA: a specially formulated Spleen qi tonic

MONTHS 2 AND 3

- ACUPUNCTURE: two or three times per week
- CLINIC FORMULA: Opioid Brain Tonic (page 198)
- OTHER CLINIC FORMULAS: specially formulated Liver and Spleen qi tonics
- SUPPLEMENTS: amino acid blend of L-tryptophan and 5-HTP, L-tyrosine, and DL-phenylalanine (DLPA) at the recommended doses listed on the product label for 6 weeks

MONTHS 3 TO 6

- ACUPUNCTURE: once or twice per week
- CLINIC FORMULAS: specially formulated Liver and Spleen qi tonics

ONGOING SELF-TREATMENT

- ACUPRESSURE: two or three times per day on points HT 7 and HT 8 (page 64), PER 7 and PER 8 (page 64), SP 3 and SP 6 (page 65), LV 2 and LV 3 (page 63), and ST 36 (page 65)
- ESSENTIAL OILS: any of those correlating to the Earth element, including coriander (page 105), fennel (page 107), or marjoram (page 112)
- MEDITATION: Five Element Meditation (page 28) twice per day

After the fifth acupuncture treatment, Sarah began coming to her sessions on her own; this signified progress to me. Her anxiety levels lessened, but this was partly since she was back living comfortably at home with her parents. Nevertheless, it took a full 3 months for her to wean off the opioids. She had begun to eat regularly and put on weight, but the eating disorder would take 8 months to 1 year to resolve, as its causes were based on events that occurred at the very beginning of her life. With 6 months of regular treatment, herbal therapy, and other complementary modalities, Sarah made the bold move of getting a job and a small studio apartment. Her root imbalances were far from resolved, but her new job was 40 miles away. After she relocated, I never heard from her again.

Metal/Lung Imbalances

The Metal element is related to our personal boundaries; a person who has had those limits broken in early childhood often has dominant Metal characteristics. Many studies have suggested that there is a strong association between abuse (physical or sexual) and addiction. Most often, the abuse began in childhood.[144] Abuse in this light may be seen as a trigger for a Metal imbalance that results in opioid dependency.

Grief is the emotion most closely associated with the Metal element, and people who have emotionally based addictions related to this element may have failed to progress through all of the stages of grief after a loss and will appear to be sad much of the time.

People with this persona type will often present with a very rigid set of beliefs and will have trouble letting go of their dogma even if it is not logical or sensible and no longer serves them well. They may also regard structure and order to such a degree that they are impossible to placate, often being referred to as perfectionists who are critically judgmental of others. Interpersonal rigor, along with addiction and its complications, creates more loss and grief as friends and family distance themselves.

The Metal element correlates to the organ systems of the Lungs and the Large Intestine. The Lungs are a major pathway of detoxification; through our breath, we eliminate toxins that do not nurture or benefit us. On a physical level, a Lung imbalance may correlate with breathing problems and detoxification issues. On an emotional level, a person with Metal attributes may be unable to let go of negative emotions.

As the brain heals during recovery from opioid dependency, people with dominant Metal characteristics will draw strength from their ability to think logically and avoid conflict and chaos. They begin to regain trust of loved ones and form new friendships because of their innate integrity and ability to be fair. As they learn how to release obsolete expectations and motivations, they are able to act with methodical efficiency in rebuilding their lives.

Lung Qi Deficiency

Lung imbalances generally arise when the Lungs do not receive enough qi to adequately perform their functions, resulting in physical and emotional issues. The Lungs are vulnerable to damp accumulations; these can be caused by Spleen qi deficiency and internal dampness (see page 41) or from external pathogens causing dampness. Another common issue seen with opioid dependency recovery is heat in the lungs, or lung yin deficiency, caused by cigarette smoking.

Self-Treatment Options for Lung Qi Deficiency

CLINIC FORMULA: Restore Lung Tonic (page 167)

PATENT FORMULA: *xiao yao san*

ACUPRESSURE POINTS: KI 6 (page 62), LU 7 and LU 9 (page 66)

SINGLE HERBS: elecampane (page 84), mullein (page 90), schisandra (page 93)

ESSENTIAL OILS: any of those correlating to the Metal element, including cypress (page 106), marjoram (page 112), or thyme (page 114)

Follow the suggestions for supporting the immune system (page 207)

RESTORE LUNG TONIC

This formula restores Lung function through the use of esteemed Lung tonic herbs. It is generally cooling if Lung heat is present and aids with the elimination of phlegm. For dosages, follow the recommendation of your licensed practitioner.

CHINESE NAME	ENGLISH NAME	PERCENTAGE OF FORMULA
Kuan dong hua	Tussilago	13.9%
Xuan fu hua	Inula flower	13.5%
Sang bai pi	Mulberry bark	13.1%
Hou po	Magnolia bark	12.7%
Su zi	Perilla seed	11.6%
Dang shen	Codonopsis	8.2%
Shan yao	Dioscorea	7.9%
Wu wei zi	Schisandra	7.5%
Tian hua fen	Trichosanthes root	5.6%
Gan jiang	Ginger (dried)	4.5%
Chen pi (ju pi)	Citrus peel (mature)	1.5%

Metal Element Imbalance
PATIENT: Justin T., male, 28 years old

After returning from Afghanistan with a traumatic brain injury (TBI), post-traumatic stress disorder (PTSD), and a leg injury from an improvised explosive device, Justin was prescribed opioid medications to control the pain. Following studies verifying that acupuncture is effective at treating symptoms related to TBI/PTSD,[145] the U.S. Veterans Administration (VA) began reimbursing for acupuncture treatments through veterans' health coverage plans.[146] More recently, studies showing the effectiveness for chronic pain due to traumatic injury have garnered even further acceptance of acupuncture.[147] During a 2011 study of the VA, it was revealed that veterans are twice as likely to die from accidental opioid overdoses as nonveterans; with this revelation, the VA began cutting back on opioid prescriptions and began to recommend alternative treatments such as acupuncture.[148] Therefore, Justin was referred to me by his local VA.

Understandably, my first impression of Justin was that he seemed quite sad. He entered the office with the aid of a cane; his leg had been saved but was permanently disfigured. He briefly described the explosion, his treatments and surgeries, and the resulting symptoms. In addition to constant pain in his leg, he suffered from headaches, flashbacks, decreased cognition, and memory loss. Without looking directly at me, he reluctantly confessed to daily crying fits. The telling of his plight filled me with a sense of urgency; this young man needed quick and effective relief from not only pain but also mental suffering.

During each acupuncture session, Justin opened up to me a bit more. He described a difficult childhood with a broken home and an absentee father. Describing himself as a "weakling," he said he was susceptible to frequent colds and suffered with childhood asthma. He had joined the military right after high school. It was a good fit for him, as he appreciated the structure of military life and had an affinity for discipline. He served for 6 years prior to the incident, and he mentioned on more than one occasion that his happiest memories were of that time. Upon returning to the States, he had felt a sense of low self-esteem when he was unable to procure regular employment. Additionally, he had not been able to form new friendships since leaving the camaraderie of the military. All of this, especially the abandonment by his father, pointed to a propensity toward Metal element imbalances.

In addition to treating points along the affected acupuncture channels related to his pain, I was also keen to focus on Lung acupuncture points during each session, because the Lung is the yin organ system associated with the Metal element. Like loss, grief, and an absentee father figure, PTSD is closely related to the Metal element, which works to reinforce personal boundaries: a traumatic attack severs the victim's integrity of self. I combined the Lung points with auricular (ear) acupuncture points for PTSD and detoxing, scalp acupuncture for brain trauma, and the Heart source point to connect Justin with his innate joy. Luckily, Justin's VA doctor worked with him to scale down the opioid medications over several months. This allowed us to build up a great amount of momentum through the acupuncture efforts, and Justin suffered no symptoms of withdrawal or increased pain during the transition.

The Treatment Protocol
WEEKS 1 TO 3

- ACUPUNCTURE: two or three times per week
- CLINIC FORMULAS FOR WITHDRAWAL: Quell Quease (page 175), Calm Mind (page 176), and Ease Detox (page 177)

WEEK 4 TO MONTH 5

- ACUPUNCTURE: two times per week
- CLINIC FORMULAS: Opioid Liver Balancer (page 150) and Opioid Brain Tonic (page 198)

ONGOING SELF-TREATMENT

- ACUPRESSURE: two or three times per day on points KI 6 (page 62), GB 41 (page 63), HT 6 (page 64), and LU 7 and LU 9 (page 66)

- ESSENTIAL OILS: any of those correlating to the Metal element, including anise seed (page 101), nutmeg (page 113), or thyme (page 114)
- MEDITATION: Five Element Meditation (page 28) twice per day

Justin's free schedule and the fact that the VA was paying for his treatment resulted in excellent compliance. He attended acupuncture sessions for 5 months until he relocated. During that time, his headaches, crying fits, and flashbacks abated, and he felt he could concentrate better. The most encouraging report was that he began volunteering most days at a youth center. He planned to move and promised to visit a community acupuncture clinic to which I referred him when he reached his new destination.

CHAPTER 8

Withdrawal
Managing Symptoms

The initial withdrawal from opioids can be challenging, even for those who have been using them as prescribed for a relatively short duration, such as a few months.[149] Opioid withdrawal syndrome, as it's known, is an indication of dependency and manifests when opioid use is discontinued. It encompasses an assortment of symptoms from nausea and vomiting to anxiety, cravings, sweating, sleep disruption, and muscle spasms. Those symptoms can range from mildly uncomfortable to positively debilitating.

The mechanisms and symptoms of withdrawal can undermine the physical capacity, energy reserves, and long-term health of anyone attempting to overcome an opioid dependency. As the alarmingly high rates of relapse show, current clinical therapies are inadequate to ensure success. Natural holistic therapies like the ones discussed in this book optimize the potential of medical interventions by supporting the physical body, building up qi (energy), and bolstering shen (spirit).

Withdrawal from opioids is only the first step in a long process of achieving sobriety and wellness. However, it can be the stumbling block that prevents progress. The importance of a successful withdrawal cannot be overstated; it sets the stage for recovery and avoidance of relapse.

Keeping these parameters in mind, health-care professionals can use natural therapies to construct realistic treatment plans for opioid users rather than simply suggesting abstinence.

Plan for Success

Before you attempt to give up opioids, it is important to make preparations, because it is unlikely that you will have the presence of mind to effectively strategize about natural therapies while in full withdrawal. Building a team of health-care professionals to support your efforts is critical.

Acupuncturist. Acupuncture will help with the physical and emotional symptoms of withdrawal, and will help prevent relapses. If possible, meet with the acupuncturist and experience a treatment prior to the withdrawal process. Two to three treatments per week are recommended at first. Look for a community acupuncture clinic in your area to reduce the cost of treatment. The benefits of a private-practice acupuncture visit include lifestyle guidance, with dietary and supplemental prescriptions. You can go to Acufinder.com to find an acupuncturist who specializes in emotional balancing and/or addiction recovery.

M.D. If you have been taking opioids by prescription, let your prescribing doctor know about your intention to stop taking them. He or she may be willing to help you with a tapering schedule. Even if you have been using opioids that were not prescribed by a doctor, your M.D. may be willing to help you with a step-down program. If not, it is advisable to have some type of professional health-care support during withdrawal, if possible.

Meditation and mindfulness instructor. Not to be underestimated, meditation can calm the mind even when you're experiencing intense stress or anxiety. Find a class, whether locally or online, and begin practicing meditation immediately so that you have established a routine before you enter withdrawal.

Nutritionist/naturopathic doctor. If you are not receiving nutritional guidance through your acupuncturist, a nutritionist can recommend supplementation, such as amino acids, that will help your brain fully recover from opioid use. In addition to arranging your treatments, you will want to purchase any herbs, dietary supplements, and pain remedies you might need ahead of time. Nutrition is critical for regaining proper brain function after opioid use. Plan as many healthy meals as you can; you can prepare some meals ahead of time and freeze them for convenience.

Weaning Off versus Quitting Cold Turkey

Weaning off opioids — that is, gradually tapering off your consumption — is preferable to sudden cessation. If you have been taking prescribed opioids, your prescribing doctor may be able to help you set up a schedule for weaning. Or your doctor may be able to prescribe opioid replacement drugs, which have a similar but milder effect to opioids in binding to opioid receptor sites in the brain; they prevent the high associated with opioid use and also minimize withdrawal symptoms.

Whether or not you are planning to use pharmaceutical assistance during the withdrawal phase, adjunct natural therapies can assist in the process, easing withdrawal symptoms and beginning the process of rebuilding health.

Some recovery programs advocate for a cold turkey approach to addiction — that is, just giving up the drugs, at once and for good. This can be very painful and is often unsuccessful. However, I have assisted countless individuals in immediate withdrawal with few, if any, side effects by implementing herbal therapy (as described in this chapter) and acupuncture four times per week.

CAUTION: AVOID INTERACTIONS WITH OPIOID REPLACEMENT DRUGS

If you are taking an opioid replacement drug like Suboxone or methadone as part of an addiction treatment program, do not use herbal therapy simultaneously. Very few studies have examined possible interactions between these drugs and herbs, and the herbs may interfere with the efficacy and dosing considerations of the medications.[150] In these cases, acupuncture therapy is the best natural therapy option to support withdrawal and recovery. Once you are no longer taking the medications, you can begin herbal therapy to support your body in its recovery of health and balance.

Getting through Withdrawal: Three Primary Formulas

A successful treatment strategy must address the symptoms that arise during the withdrawal stage. I use three main clinic formulas with multiple modes of action. These three formulas are most commonly all taken together during the first 5 to 7 days of withdrawal to address the debilitating symptoms that most often lead people to abandon the treatment protocols and relapse into opioid use.

You will want to have these formulas on hand before beginning withdrawal from opioids to ensure a smooth transition. Planning your strategies and preparing for treatment protocols is key to success. You, whether as caretaker or patient, do not want to be in full panic mode and trying to procure herbs in the midst of withdrawal.

OPIOID WITHDRAWAL FORMULA 1: QUELL QUEASE

This formula contains potent herbs that ease nausea and vomiting. It is not a tonic formula to be used over a long period of time for chronic nausea; the clinic formula Opioid Spleen Tonic (page 161) would be better for that purpose. This Quell Quease formula is often taken first thing in the morning so that the patient can better tolerate other herb formulas and foods without queasiness. It can be difficult to keep anything in your stomach during the acute withdrawal stage.

Take this formula with a cup of warm broth. For dosages, follow the recommendation of your licensed practitioner.

CHINESE NAME	ENGLISH NAME	PERCENTAGE OF FORMULA
Cang zhu	Atractylodes	11.4%
Huo xiang	Agastache	11.3%
Shen qu	Massa medicata	11.1%
Shan zha	Crataegus	7.3%
Yi yi ren	Coix	7.1%
Fu ling	Poria	6.9%
Ju hong	Red tangerine peel	5.6%
Xiang fu	Cyperus rhizome	5.6%
Da zao (hong)	Jujube dates (red)	5.6%
Tian hua fen	Trichosanthes root	5.6%
Mu xiang	Vladimiria	5.6%
Ge gen	Pueraria root	5.6%
Gu ya	Rice or millet sprout (oryza)	5.6%
Ban xia (zhi)	Pinellia	1.9%
Mai men dong	Ophiopogon	1.9%
Hou po	Magnolia bark	1.9%

OPIOID WITHDRAWAL FORMULA 2: CALM MIND

This potent herb formula calms the mind, or shen. It can alleviate anxiety, panic attacks, and cravings and help one get to sleep, as sleep and stress issues are pronounced during withdrawal. The formula can be used throughout the day as prescribed, but it is especially helpful if taken at around 9:00 p.m. to ready the mind for sleep. It can be taken for up to 3 months while the body and mind work to balance out. Once any root organ system imbalances are addressed, the mind will begin to self-regulate. For dosages, follow the recommendation of your licensed practitioner.

CHINESE NAME	ENGLISH NAME	PERCENTAGE OF FORMULA
He huan pi	Albizzia bark	17.2%
Bai shao	Peony (white)	12.0%
Long gu (duan)	Dragon bone (fossil)	9.9%
He shou wu	Fo-ti	9.4%
Bai zi ren	Biota seed	8.6%
Yuan zhi	Polygala	7.3%
Che qian zi	Plantago seed	6.9%
Zhen zhu mu	Mother of pearl	6.4%
Fu shen	Poria	5.6%
Wu wei zi	Schisandra	5.2%
Dang gui (shen)	Dong gui	4.7%
Mu li (duan)	Oyster shell (calcined)	4.3%
Suan zao ren	Zizyphus	2.1%
Hu po	Amber	0.4%

OPIOID WITHDRAWAL FORMULA 3: EASE DETOX

This herb formula quickens the detoxification of opioids from the body utilizing herbs that stimulate Liver detoxification and Lymphatic drainage. It effectively breaks up Liver qi stagnation, which would contribute to muscle cramps/spasms and sleep disruptions. Detoxification herbs are generally quite cooling in nature, and this formula helps ease the sweats associated with the acute withdrawal period. It is meant to be used during the first 2 to 3 weeks of withdrawal. For dosages, follow the recommendation of your licensed practitioner.

CHINESE NAME	ENGLISH NAME	PERCENTAGE OF FORMULA
Xuan shen	Scrophularia	11.1%
Bai shao	Peony (white)	8.9%
Xia ku cao	Spica prunellae	8.6%
Tian hua fen	Trichosanthes root	8.3%
Bai ji li	Tribulus	8.0%
Zhi mu	Anemarrhena rhizome	6.4%
Dan zhu ye	Lophatherum	6.1%
Da qing ye	Isatis leaf	5.8%
Gou teng	Gambir	5.5%
Xiang fu	Cyperus rhizome	5.3%
Chai hu	Bupleurum	5.0%
Shi jue ming	Abalone shell (haliotis)	4.2%
Han lian cao	Eclipta	3.3%
Qing pi	Citrus peel (green)	2.8%
Fang feng	Siler	2.5%
Pu gong ying	Dandelion	2.2%
Zhi zi (shan)	Gardenia	1.9%
Bai zi ren	Biota seed	1.7%
Dan shen	Salvia root	1.1%
Dang gui (shen)	Dong gui	0.8%
Suan zao ren	Zizyphus	0.6%

Self-Treatment Options

We'll look at some self-treatment options for the common symptoms of withdrawal, but in my experience, these patent formulas, herbs, and other treatments are not targeted for withdrawal and are not as strong acting as the primary clinic formulas given previously. That being said, these options can be quite helpful if you are left with no other choice, and they can complement the primary formulas.

SELF-TREATMENT OPTIONS FOR NAUSEA AND VOMITING

PATENT FORMULA: *tai kang ning*

SINGLE HERBS: hawthorn (page 86), meadowsweet (page 89); ginger and peppermint would also help

ESSENTIAL OILS: any of those correlating to the Earth element, including coriander (page 105) or fennel (page 107)

ACUPRESSURE POINTS: SP 3, SP 6, SP 9, ST 36 (page 65)

SELF-TREATMENT OPTIONS FOR ANXIETY AND CRAVINGS

PATENT FORMULA: *an shen bu xin*

SINGLE HERBS: lavender (page 88), lemon balm (page 88), reishi (page 92), schisandra (page 93), skullcap (page 94)

ESSENTIAL OILS: any of those correlating to the Fire element, including clary sage (page 104), ho wood (page 110), or lavender (page 110)

ACUPRESSURE POINTS: HT 7, HT 8, PER 6, PER 7 (page 64)

SELF-TREATMENT OPTIONS TO HASTEN DETOX

PATENT FORMULAS: *long dan xie gan pian plus tian ma gou teng pian*

SINGLE HERBS: dandelion (page 83), yellow dock (page 97); other good options would be cleavers, nettle, or plantain

ESSENTIAL OILS: basil (page 102), cypress (page 106), or Mandarin Orange/Tangerine (page 111)

ACUPRESSURE POINTS: LV 2, LV 3, GB 41 (page 63), LI 4, LI 11 (page 66)

CURING PILLS/TAI KANG NING

The popular patent formula *tai kang ning* was rightly named Curing Pills because it is able to address such a wide array of digestive complaints and conditions. Curing Pills have traditionally been used for any type of acute digestive disorder, including indigestion from overeating, nausea associated with weak digestion, vomiting due to stomach flu, diarrhea associated with food poisoning, gas, and acid reflux. In cases of withdrawal from opioids, Curing Pills have been shown to be as effective as lofexidine, a medication commonly prescribed to alleviate the symptoms of withdrawal from heroin and other opioids.[151]

Muscle Cramps and Spasms

Researchers have now spent decades trying to decipher the mechanisms underlying opioid withdrawal symptoms, without great success. Some theorize that the symptoms arise from multiple neurotransmitters acting on many different receptor sites in both the central and peripheral nervous systems.[152] Among the mysterious symptoms of withdrawal are muscle cramping, spasms, and restless leg syndrome. From the perspective of traditional Chinese medicine, these are due to internal wind caused by Liver qi stagnation, which creates Liver heat. In ancient times, Liver fire typically arose from pathogenic diseases such as hemorrhagic fever; in modern times, Liver heat is more commonly related to drug and/or alcohol consumption, poor dietary practices, and emotional stresses. The condition actually develops over a long time, but the Liver heat can result in muscle spasms very quickly upon withdrawal because of the cessation of the opioid drug that has been preventing the physical muscle cramps. This can result in great discomfort and loss of sleep. Luckily, clearing heat with acupuncture and detoxifying herbs will help alleviate these symptoms.

CHAPTER 9

Pain

Using Natural Therapies
in Place of Narcotics

Opioid prescriptions for treating pain that arises from injuries, illnesses, and aging are one avenue by which we have arrived at a national opioid epidemic. An often-cited 2013 study reported that 80 percent of heroin users had used prescription painkillers before turning to heroin,[153] and similar statistics have led many states to enact new laws limiting opioid use.[154] These regulations, along with fear of developing addiction, have left many people suffering from pain in a precarious position and searching for alternatives.

Treating pain effectively without the use of opioid medications and reducing the duration of time for which patients require prescription painkillers are two factors directly relevant to the opioid epidemic. So how can we treat pain without narcotics? Acupuncture, in conjunction with herbs and natural topical remedies, may be the answer. Countless studies have concluded that acupuncture helps to manage chronic and acute pain.[155] Furthermore, acupuncture has been proved to be an effective analgesic for postoperative pain, thus reducing the need for opioid medication and reducing the risk of opioid dependency developing.[156]

Acupuncture is the optimal nonpharmacological option for pain management, but there are others, and what works for each of us will differ based on our constitution and the etiology of the pain we experience. In this chapter, we will discuss several natural strategies for pain management. But please note: if you are experiencing acute pain or intractable chronic pain, seek the help of a qualified medical practitioner.

Natural versus Pharmaceutical Pain Therapies

When using herbs for pain relief, you are working with the body to increase circulation and reduce inflammation; this is much different from medications that block pain receptor sites in the brain. Herbs work with your body to bring true healing, and true healing takes time. A comparison could be made with high blood pressure. Western medicine treats high blood pressure with medications like diuretics and beta blockers, which have rapid effects. TCM treats high blood pressure with herbs, acupuncture, and other modalities. The Chinese method takes effect over many months, rather than right away, but it treats the actual underlying imbalances in the body at a very deep level.

Likewise, acupuncture works to address the true causes of imbalance that lead to symptoms of ill health. You wouldn't go to physical therapy and expect just one session to resolve your pain, but many people have such expectations for acupuncture. From time to time, a single acupuncture session will have immediate, lasting results, but this is the exception rather than the rule. Depending on the severity of the condition, a course of treatment is typically noted as 10 consecutive sessions. An acute minor injury might respond more quickly; a serious or chronic injury might take longer. I am always flabbergasted when a new patient comes in saying, "I thought I would give acupuncture a try to see if it works," expecting results in one treatment. My patients often experience immediate pain relief during their first session, but I explain that the pain might return in a day or two. With each session, the episodes of pain become less frequent.

The typical recovery involves gradual improvement, with the nature and intensity of the pain easing up and the bouts of pain occurring less often. I expect some change, which includes the location of the pain, within three to six sessions. During treatments I often ask patients, "Where is your pain now?" This is because of the way the brain perceives pain. While you may have multiple areas producing pain, the brain can process only a limited number of pain neurons.[157] Therefore, when acupuncture clears pain in one area the patient senses pain in another area. Patients believe that the pain has "moved," but in reality, the strongest pain sensation has been eliminated and a previously weaker one can now be felt. The patient must change the black-and-white perception of "I have pain, or I do not" to "My pain syndrome is gradually changing and lessening."

Compared to natural medicine, opioids are faster and more efficient at eliminating pain. However, long-term use of opioids is rarely sustainable and opioid toxins are damaging the body the entire time they are administered. TCM therapies are slower to resolve pain but are actually healing the body and have few, if any, negative side effects. The two strategies cannot be compared like for like. Opioids are a sledgehammer, whereas natural remedies are a soft whisper that reminds the body how to heal itself.

Therefore, when relying on gentle, natural remedies to heal, full compliance and a strong commitment are necessary for great outcomes. Patients will sometimes come into my clinic stating that they just want acupuncture and not herbal therapy, that they just want herbs and not acupuncture, or that they do not have time to improve their lifestyle habits or meditate. Each exclusion from their treatment protocol lessens their chances of a good outcome and increases their cost and length of therapy. While each person who works to transition away from opioid dependency will have a unique healing strategy, you will want to consistently use as many natural modalities as possible. You must also accept that this therapy is going to take many months.

Stagnation Causes Pain

In TCM theory, pain results from qi stagnation and/or blood stagnation. As we've discussed, qi is the vital energy that circulates through our meridians. When qi is blocked or sluggish, stagnation results. Burning or tingling pain, like the kind associated with nerve pain, is often attributed to qi stagnation.

Blood stagnation can result from qi stagnation, or it can result from injury or trauma such as cuts, wounds, bruises, or sprains. Pain resulting from blood stagnation tends to be sharp and fixed. As it turns out, blood goes where qi goes, so the two are typically seen together.

We use herbs and acupuncture to break up qi and blood stagnation, clear heat and toxins that contributed to the stagnation, and restore balance to the body, thus healing the underlying cause of pain.

SELF-TREATMENT OPTIONS FOR PAIN

- PATENT FORMULA: *yunnan bai yao*

- SINGLE HERBS: cannabis (page 82), meadowsweet (page 89), wild lettuce (page 95)

- Topical herb remedies (page 185)

- ORGAN SUPPORT: tonic herbs associated with the organ system that governs the type of pain you're experiencing

- ACUPRESSURE POINTS: LI 4 (page 66) combined with LV 3 (page 63), and any points along the meridian associated with the organ system that governs the type of pain you're experiencing (see page 29)

BONE BREAK FORMULA

This herb formula is based on an ancient remedy for trauma and chronic pain. It has many actions, including moving blood and qi. It supports the Kidneys and so is ideal for back pain. In Chinese medicine, nourishing marrow is part of the process of "bone knitting," and this formula

CHINESE NAME	ENGLISH NAME	PERCENTAGE OF FORMULA
Gu sui bu	Drynaria	6.7%
Mu xiang (chuang)	Vladimiria	6.7%
Jiang huang	Turmeric	6.4%
Xu duan	Dipsacus	6.4%
Liu ji nu	Artemisiae anomalae	6.2%
Wu jia pi	Acanthopanax giraldii	5.9%
Mo yao (duan)	Myrrh	5.5%
Ru xiang (duan)	Mastic	5.5%
Lu lu tong	Liquidambar	5.5%
Chi shao	Peony (red)	5.2%
Su mu	Sappan wood	5.0%
Yan hu suo	Corydalis	4.0%
Mu dan pi (su)	Moutan	3.8%
Chuan xiong	Ligusticum	3.6%
Bai shao	Peony (white)	3.3%
Chen pi (ju pi)	Citrus peel (mature)	3.3%
Tao ren	Peach kernel (persica)	3.1%
Jie geng	Platycodon	3.1%
Dang gui (shen)	Dong gui	2.9%
Zhi shi	Aurantium immaturus	2.9%
Fang feng	Siler	2.6%
San leng	Scirpus	2.4%

includes herbs to do just that. The name of the formula honors its origins; whether you have a broken bone or not, these potent tonic herbs will speed healing. It is also appropriate for chronic pain conditions. It would be taken for 6 weeks to 3 months in cases of acute trauma, and longer for chronic pain. Note that this formula should not be started until serious injuries with bleeding are contained. For dosages, follow the recommendation of your licensed practitioner.

Topical Remedies for Pain Due to Trauma

Topical treatment for pain resulting from trauma or injury — everything from bruises and sprains to broken bones and surgical incisions — can be divided into three stages:

- STAGE 1: the first and second days after injury

- STAGE 2: the first 2 weeks after injury

- STAGE 3: the third week to the sixth week after injury

Each stage has its own mode of action to minimize pain and enhance healing.

Stage 1: Days 1 to 2

Immediately following trauma, we typically experience swelling at the site of injury. This swelling can cause tissue damage beyond that attributed to the traumatic event itself. However, according to Chinese medical theory, applying actual ice to the injury prevents and/or delays healing. Instead, Chinese practitioners use "herbal ice" — a blend of herbs that are cold in nature yet stimulate blood flow so that lymphatic fluids are not constricted and impeded from assisting with the healing process. While the classic formula on page 186 does contain astringents that reduce bleeding when applied topically, it mostly focuses on lessening swelling.

Herbal Ice

Apply this cooling herbal spray to injuries as soon as they occur. This is an important remedy to stock in your first-aid kit, as it is time-consuming to make, and it is meant to be applied immediately following trauma.

INGREDIENTS

- ⅛ ounce Chinese skullcap (*Scutellaria baicalensis*) root
- ⅛ ounce dandelion root
- ⅛ ounce gysum
- ⅛ ounce gardenia flower
- ⅛ ounce Oregon grape root
- ⅛ ounce phellodendron root bark
- ⅛ ounce rhubarb root
- ⅛ ounce safflower flower
- 2 cups 80-proof vodka
- ¼ teaspoon green mandarin (qing pi) essential oil
- ¼ teaspoon litsea essential oil
- ¼ teaspoon peppermint essential oil

PREPARATION

Grind the dry herbs in a dedicated coffee grinder. Place the dry herb powder on a baking pan and lightly brown in an oven set to broil, stirring often. Then place the dry herb material in a glass mason jar and cover with the vodka. Seal the jar and shake the contents for 2 minutes. Shake the contents for 2 minutes each day for 2 weeks. Strain the herbs, squeezing all the liquid through a cheesecloth; wrap the herb leavings in the cheesecloth and set aside. Add the essential oils to the prepared tincture and pour into a glass spray bottle for application. Shake prior to each application. Can store up to 2 years.

USE

Apply every waking hour or two immediately following a sprain, strain, or other traumatic injury at the site of impact during the first 2 days of recovery to lessen swelling. Save the cheesecloth-wrapped herbs in a sealed container to use as a compress.

LAYING RICE TO REST

Rest, ice, compression, and elevation (RICE) has been the standard treatment for athletic injuries in Western medicine since 1978, when Dr. Gabe Mirkin coined the acronym. But Chinese medicine has never accepted this treatment protocol as productive. As a matter of fact, TCM considers the RICE method a mistreatment of traumatic injuries that can lead to long-term pain, arthritis, and reduced mobility.

Ice constricts the flow of blood and lymph fluid and thereby slows swelling. The thinking behind the RICE method was that it would lessen tissue damage. However, studies have found that the practice of icing, while it reduces inflammation, actually delays the recovery of damaged muscles.[158] The same is true of anti-inflammatory pain relievers such as ibuprofen. Even Dr. Mirkin now publicly questions the first-aid method that he originally advocated. He now suggests icing for no more than 10 minutes, with at least 20 minutes between ice sessions. He also suggests that ice treatment continue for no more than 6 hours after the injury.[159]

Stage 2: Weeks 1 to 2

In this phase of recovery, you've handled the immediate requirements of trauma, and now you are ready to use herbs to remove stagnation, swelling, and toxic heat. Warm herbal soaks and hot packs would not be appropriate at this time, because you want to get rid of heat, not add to it.

Heat-Clearing Trauma Spray

Use this blend after any initial swelling has been resolved by the Herbal Ice formula (page 186). It is safe to use on broken skin, but be warned, the alcohol in the spray will burn a bit. Yarrow and cattail pollen are used to stop bleeding, while other herbs such as dong quai, frankincense, red peony, and red sage move blood and encourage healing and prevent stagnation.

INGREDIENTS

¼ ounce yarrow leaf and flower

⅛ ounce Aucklandia root

⅛ ounce black cohosh root

⅛ ounce cattail pollen

⅛ ounce clove flower bud

⅛ ounce dong quai root

⅛ ounce frankincense resin

⅛ ounce gardenia flower

⅛ ounce myrrh gum

⅛ ounce peach seeds

⅛ ounce red peony root

⅛ ounce red sage root

⅛ ounce rhubarb root

⅛ ounce safflower flower

⅛ ounce white mulberry twig

4 cups 80-proof vodka

½ teaspoon Atlas cedar essential oil

½ teaspoon camphor essential oil

½ teaspoon green mandarin (qing pi) essential oil

½ teaspoon litsea essential oil

½ teaspoon peppermint essential oil

PREPARATION

Grind the dry herbs in a coffee grinder. Place the dry herb powder on a baking pan and lightly brown in an oven set to broil, stirring often. Then place the dry herb material in a glass mason jar and cover with the vodka. Seal the jar and shake the contents for 2 minutes. Shake the contents for 2 minutes each day for 2 weeks. Strain the herbs, squeezing all the liquid through a cheesecloth; wrap the herb leavings in the cheesecloth and set aside. Add the essential oils to the prepared tincture and pour into a glass spray bottle for application. Shake prior to each application. Can store up to 2 years.

USE

Following Herbal Ice (page 186), apply this spray to the site of injury five or six times per day and allow to air-dry to lessen pain and speed recovery. Follow with Warming Recovery Spray (page 190) for a full recovery. Save the cheesecloth-wrapped herbs in a sealed container to use as a compress.

Stage 3: Weeks 3 to 6

Now warming essential oils, herbs, and wet heat can be used to nourish the tendons and make sure that tissue adhesions, which will result in stiffness, do not develop. If appropriate, gentle movement can help speed healing at this stage.

Warming Recovery Spray

This warming spray will assist in healing not only new injuries but also old injuries that were not addressed correctly and now cause pain with cold weather. It is not appropriate for red, swollen, inflamed areas; reserve it for use on injuries that have passed through the swelling phase or chronic areas of pain such as cold, stiff joints. This formula should not be applied to broken skin.

INGREDIENTS

¼ ounce arnica flowers

¼ ounce yarrow leaf and flower

⅛ ounce Aucklandia root

⅛ ounce black cohosh root

⅛ ounce club moss herb

⅛ ounce dong quai root

⅛ ounce frankincense resin

⅛ ounce mulberry twig

⅛ ounce myrrh gum

⅛ ounce peach seeds

⅛ ounce red peony root

⅛ ounce red sage root

⅛ ounce safflower flower

4 cups 80-proof vodka

¼ teaspoon Atlas cedar essential oil

¼ teaspoon camphor essential oil

¼ teaspoon cinnamon essential oil

¼ teaspoon ginger essential oil

¼ teaspoon green mandarin (qing pi) essential oil

¼ teaspoon rosemary essential oil

¼ teaspoon star anise essential oil

¼ teaspoon sweet marjoram essential oil

PREPARATION

Grind the dry herbs in a coffee grinder. Place the dry herb powder on a baking pan and lightly brown in an oven set to broil, stirring often. Then place the dry herb material in a glass mason jar and cover with the vodka. Seal the jar and shake the contents for 2 minutes. Shake the contents for 2 minutes each day for 2 weeks. Strain the herbs, squeezing all the liquid through a cheesecloth; wrap the herb leavings in the cheesecloth and set aside. Add the essential oils to the prepared tincture and pour into a glass spray bottle for application. Shake prior to each application. Can store up to 2 years.

USE

Apply four to six times per day during weeks 3 to 6 after injury, as needed, to lessen pain and speed recovery. Save the cheesecloth-wrapped herbs in a sealed container to use as a compress.

VARIATIONS

As we discussed in chapter 5, essential oils correspond to specific organ systems and the correlating meridians. Anise seed essential oil, for example, corresponds to the Liver, Spleen, Stomach, and Lungs. You can add essential oils that target specific areas of pain to the Warming Recovery Spray to target the formula and open the specific meridians where qi and blood stagnation are causing pain.

Chronic Pain and Stiffness Due to Dampness

If an injury is not addressed correctly and in a timely manner in stages 1, 2, and 3, dampness or phlegm may develop, making prolonged pain a probability. The strategies described earlier in this chapter must continue to be employed while dampness is purged from the tissue and joints. If dampness develops, expect recovery to take many months. Pain due to internal dampness is referred to as damp bi (*bi*, pronounced "bee," simply means pain in Chinese medicine).

Internal dampness can develop when the body does not manage fluids well, likely due to Spleen qi deficiency. This type of pain tends to be deep and dull pain in the muscles or joints, and is aggravated with wet weather, rain, humid climate, or damp conditions. This type of pain would likely be deep, achy, muscular pain with a heavy feeling in the body, and there can be episodes of hot, swollen joints. Viscous, sticky internal dampness blocks the free flow of qi and blood.

Damp Bi Spray

Apply this spray topically to help resolve pain due to internal dampness forming in the muscle tissue and joints.

INGREDIENTS

½ ounce barberry

½ ounce Job's tears

⅛ ounce *Angelica pubescens*

⅛ ounce Aucklandia root

⅛ ounce black cohosh root

⅛ ounce dang gui

⅛ ounce fang feng root

⅛ ounce mulberry twig

⅛ ounce peach seeds

⅛ ounce poke root

⅛ ounce prickly ash bark

⅛ ounce red peony root

⅛ ounce red sage root

⅛ ounce rhubarb root

⅛ ounce safflower flower

⅛ ounce St. John's wort

⅛ ounce yarrow leaf and flower

6 cups 80-proof vodka

¼ teaspoon Atlas cedar essential oil

¼ teaspoon black pepper essential oil

¼ teaspoon camphor essential oil

¼ teaspoon cinnamon essential oil

¼ teaspoon ginger root essential oil

¼ teaspoon guiac wood essential oil

¼ teaspoon Himalayan cedar essential oil

¼ teaspoon peppermint essential oil

¼ teaspoon rosemary essential oil

¼ teaspoon wintergreen essential oil

PREPARATION

Grind the dry herbs in a coffee grinder. Place the dry herb powder on a baking pan and lightly brown in an oven set to broil, stirring often. Then place the dry herb material in a glass mason jar and cover with the vodka. Seal the jar and shake the contents for 2 minutes. Shake the contents for 2 minutes each day for 2 weeks. Strain the herbs, squeezing all the liquid through a cheesecloth; wrap the herb leavings in the cheesecloth and set aside. Add the essential oils to the prepared tincture and pour into a glass spray bottle for application. Shake prior to each application. Can store up to 2 years.

USE

Apply four to six times per day as needed to lessen pain and speed recovery. Do not use on open cuts or wounds. Can be used as needed for chronic pain arising from an injury that was not addressed properly following the traumatic incident. Save the cheesecloth-wrapped herbs in a sealed container to use as a compress.

CHAPTER 10

Health Problems
Addressing the Long-Term Effects of Opioid Use

Opioid use can lead to long-term negative health effects, and these effects can persist for months or even years if not resolved appropriately. While not exhaustive, this chapter covers the more common health conditions that result from chronic use of opioids along with natural therapies that can be used to address the imbalances that lead to these disease patterns. The suggested natural therapies can typically be integrated with Western medical approaches to opioid dependency recovery.

As with any disease, the treatment plan will depend not only on the severity and the duration but also on the patient's overall health and vitality. With diabetes, for example, I would expect a patient with insulin resistance, or prediabetes, to experience complete recovery after 3 to 6 months of regular treatments with herbs, acupuncture, and nutritional therapy. Thereafter, the patient can maintain good health through good lifestyle habits, such as consuming nourishing foods and herbs, getting regular exercise and sleep, and practicing daily meditation. In contrast, patients who come into my clinic with a long history of chronic diabetes can slow the progression of the disease with natural therapies, but they will likely need to keep taking their pharmaceutical medications throughout their life.

The same can be said for opioid dependency. If the dependency is treated early on, natural therapies can reverse the negative emotional and physical impacts of the drug use. In cases of chronic addiction, patients can expect a lifelong treatment effort to maintain relative wellness, with occasional downturns in health.

Memory and Cognitive Deficits

People who experience opioid dependency can suffer from lingering cognitive deficiencies induced by neural dysregulation in the prefrontal cortex.[160] For those who have used prescription opioids as short-term pain relievers, the effects on the brain may last for only a few weeks or months. These effects may include problems with holding focus, solving complex problems, and long- or short-term memory.

However, opioid overdoses can lead to slowed or irregular breathing, loss of consciousness, brain hypoxia (insufficient oxygen reaching the brain), and other conditions that cause more serious brain damage. Those who survive may experience a variety of temporary or long-term cognitive issues:

- Problems concentrating
- Difficulty making decisions
- Memory loss
- Reduced ability to move the body

- Loss of coordination and balance
- Paralysis
- Hearing and/or vision impairment
- Inability or reduced ability to communicate, read, or write[161]

From the perspective of traditional Chinese medicine, thought, memory, and the mind are influenced by the five elements, which encompass all mental-spiritual aspects of human beings. Because Chinese medicine does not separate the body, mind, and spirit, mental and spiritual deficits and imbalances can be addressed by supporting the associated physical organs through natural therapies such as herbs, essential oils, acupressure, and so on. If you understand how cognitive capacities correlate to the the elements, you can identify which organ system is imbalanced by observing manifestations of cognitive deficits.

Water/Kidneys

Water exerts its influence over the Kidneys. They share the power of decision-making with the Liver, as they house jing, which, along with the shen, is responsible for our acquired wisdom through life. We cannot plan and make wise decisions without reflecting on past experiences and acquired knowledge. Additionally, the Kidney organ system is responsible for our willpower.

Wood/Liver

The Liver belongs to the Wood element and stores *po* (primitive memories) and *hun* (subconscious); it houses the intelligence of the cells, or our instinctual memories. The Liver empowers us to plan and envision our future. When Liver qi is not flowing well and generates heat, we lose our wisdom and can become destructive.

Fire/Heart

The Fire element relates to summer, when the toil of spring's efforts come to fruition; thus, a healthy Heart allows us to bring any plans we made through the vision of Wood energy to come to fruition and for our thoughts to fully develop.

Clear thinking depends on a strong Heart, which is the yin organ of Fire. The Heart stores the evolving consciousness, or shen, and emotional disorders of the mind are attributed to shen disorders. The shen is also responsible for our ideas, which are projected through thoughts that give our life purpose. The Heart is the only organ system able to provide insights into our emotions; the other organs cannot perceive emotional feelings.

Earth/Spleen

The Spleen is associated with the Earth element and stores *zhi* (knowledge) and *yi* (ideation). It is associated with thinking, ideas, memorization, and studying. If the Spleen is damaged, people may find that they obsess over and rehash the same thoughts over and over.

The process of learning is assigned to the Earth element. In terms of opioid dependency, if we cannot learn from past mistakes, then falling into the old patterns of imbalance that are associated with dependency is inevitable. Opioid use strongly imprints in our memories and associations with people, places, and things, which contributes to recidivism. Supporting the Earth element allows us to form new, healthy associations and memories, contributing to recovery.

Metal/Lungs

Metal corresponds to the Lungs and helps us maintain a sense of self-worth and positive boundaries. When we breathe, we take in purity in the form of oxygen and release toxins in the form of carbon dioxide. In a similar way, the Lungs work to bring in positive thoughts and release negativity. If we become polluted, mentally and spiritually, by opioid use, the Lungs may not be able to keep up with their duties. Alternatively, sometimes pollution, like abuse during our childhood, leads to Lung deficiency and a lack of self-worth, which could drive us toward opioid use. Whatever the case, the Lungs must be performing optimally before we can cleanse ourselves of old habits and beliefs and help to create a new positive vision of who we are.

SELF-TREATMENT OPTIONS FOR MEMORY AND COGNITIVE DEFICITS

- PATENT FORMULA: *bu nao*

- SINGLE HERBS: schisandra (page 93)

- ESSENTIAL OILS: basil (page 102), clary sage (page 104), or rosemary (page 113)

- ACUPRESSURE POINTS: HT 5, HT 7, HT 8, PER 6, PER 7, PER 8 (page 64), ST 36 (page 65)

OPIOID BRAIN TONIC

This formula contains tonic herbs known to enhance cognitive function. It is useful in enhancing the body's natural function of neuroplasticity and brain repair. It would be useful for anyone who has used or abused opioids and finds that their personality has changed, their motivation is lacking, or their memory is impaired. It may also be useful in fighting cravings for opioids by remodeling the brain so that it no longer draws connections between environmental triggers — people, places, and things — and drug use. Depending on the severity of cognitive deficit, you could expect to take this formula for many months to 1 year. For dosages, follow the recommendation of your licensed practitioner.

CHINESE NAME	ENGLISH NAME	PERCENTAGE OF FORMULA
Yin xing ye (yin guo ye)	Ginkgo leaf	9.4%
Nu zhen zi	Ligustrum	8.9%
Tu si zi	Cuscuta seed	8.7%
He shou wu (zhi)	Fo-ti	6.8%
Gou qi zi	Lycium fruit	6.8%
Wu wei zi	Schisandra	6.6%
Dan shen	Salvia root	6.3%
Shu di huang	Rehmannia (cooked)	6.0%
Du zhong (chao)	Eucommia (dry-fried)	5.5%
Yuan zhi	Polygala	5.2%
Mai men dong	Ophiopogon	4.5%
Tian men dong	Asparagus	4.2%
Ling zhi (red)	Ganoderma (red)	4.2%
Lu rong	Deer antler velvet	3.9%
Ren shen (hong)	Ginseng	3.9%
Dang gui (shen)	Dong gui	3.4%
Da zao (hong)	Jujube dates (red)	3.1%
Chen pi (ju pi)	Citrus peel (mature)	2.6%

Fatigue

During the initial weeks, and sometimes even months, after opioid withdrawal, many people feel intensely tired. The following sections describe some of the common patterns that can lead to fatigue.

Spleen Qi Deficiency Fatigue

Qi is formed by the food we eat and by the air we breathe. Many people addicted to opioids do not eat when they are using, and this leads to Spleen qi deficiency. One of the symptoms of Spleen insufficiencies is a poor appetite, so a cycle of imbalance can be imbedded. Once the damage is done, efforts to improve Spleen health can be difficult without the intervention of herbs and acupuncture. A healthy diverse diet including adequate protein is necessary to produce our daily energy.

To address Spleen qi deficiency, see the recommendations on page 160. To address fatigue in general, try the clinic formula Restore Energy and Vibrance (page 200).

Dampness Fatigue

The Spleen organ system oversees the transformation of foods and fluids. If the Spleen becomes congested by too much food, inappropriate foods, or foods and drinks that are cold, Spleen function will be damaged. When this happens, internal dampness develops because the Spleen is unable to perform its duty in transforming fluids throughout the body. Fatigue with internal dampness will be marked by a feeling of heaviness in the body, a heavy head with brain fog, and trouble getting going in the morning. Internal dampness and resulting fatigue of this type is treated by reinforcing the Spleen. See the discussion of the Spleen organ system (page 34) for more detail. And note that the Spleen's active time is in the early morning, so eating breakfast is pivotal in the formation of qi.

RESTORE ENERGY AND VIBRANCE

This formula contains tonic herbs that fortify qi. It is ideal for anyone going through opioid withdrawal and feeling chronically sluggish and tired. It would be used for a number of months to fortify the body until the person is able to make their own qi through a proper diet and healthy lifestyle habits such as regular exercise. It may take a few weeks before improvements are noticed. The formula does not contain stimulants, but some people have trouble getting to sleep if they take this formula too late at night; in that case, take it in the morning. For dosages, follow the recommendation of your licensed practitioner.

CHINESE NAME	ENGLISH NAME	PERCENTAGE OF FORMULA
Huang qi (bei)	Astragalus root	10.2%
Bai zhu	Atractylodes (alba)	9.8%
Bai shao	Peony (white)	9.2%
Dang shen	Codonopsis	8.9%
He shou wu (zhi)	Fo-ti	8.5%
Shu di huang	Rehmannia (cooked)	7.9%
Shan yao	Dioscorea	7.5%
Mu dan pi (su)	Moutan	6.9%
Jiao gu lan	Gynostemma	6.2%
Long yan rou	Longan fruit	5.9%
Dang gui (shen)	Dong gui	5.6%
Shan zhu yu	Cornus	5.2%
Da zao (hong)	Jujube dates (red)	4.9%
Chen pi (ju pi)	Citrus peel (mature)	3.3%

Lung Qi Deficiency Fatigue

As mentioned earlier, the lungs play a vital role in producing qi from the air we breathe and the food we consume. With lung qi deficiency, a common occurrence among opioid users (see page 35), or when there is a constriction of airflow due to asthma, chronic obstructive pulmonary disease (COPD), or emphysema, the body is unable to produce the vital energy it needs to get through the day effectively. See page 166 for recommendations on treating Lung qi deficiency.

Heart Qi Deficiency Fatigue

Qi deficiency is a common imbalance of the Heart organ system. For oxygen and nutrients to reach our organs and tissue, abundant blood must be flowing throughout our vessels. Heart qi deficiency can lead to the heart not pumping blood effectively. The resulting poor circulation leads to a lessened supply of oxygen available for cells. This oxygen is necessary for energy production in the body at a cellular level. If cells do not have oxygen, fatigue can develop. Heart qi deficiency would be marked by palpitations, poor sleep, shortness of breath, poor cognitive skills, or numbness in the extremities. See the discussion on page 155 for details on treating this imbalance.

Adrenal Fatigue

Recent studies have shown that ongoing use of drugs such as opioids leads to adrenal fatigue; this is a very common malady in recovering addicts.[162] Chinese herbs and acupuncture have been used to successfully reverse this difficult disease. While the process is not fast, TCM is one of the few modalities that can spare individuals from a lifetime of fatigue and declining health due to adrenal burnout.

The Kidneys store the jing, while qi provides our daily energy needs. Jing is a dense substance that is used sparingly throughout our life. When all jing is depleted, we die, so it is important to preserve our jing; additionally, jing is very difficult to restore. Opioids cause the body to squander and deplete the rare reserves of jing. Ongoing stress and pushing yourself too hard for too long also depletes jing. Qi deficiency can lead to fatigue, but adrenal exhaustion is much deeper.[163]

Adrenal fatigue is a classic example of Kidney deficiency exhaustion. Kidney tonic herbs and formulas like those on pages 142 to 145 work to boost your body up from within, over time. Unlike drugs and caffeine or energy drinks, tonic herbs will not give you a quick, artificial boost of energy and an adrenaline rush; stimulating the release of adrenaline in this way is often part of the cause of adrenal exhaustion. Instead, herbal tonic formulas will help rebuild what you have been depleting and restore wellness and true core vitality by restoring the organ systems.

For many people, there is a correlation between adrenal fatigue and low blood sugar, so it is important to eat good, wholesome natural and organic foods at regular intervals to avoid a drop in blood sugar, which can exacerbate your condition. One of the best things you can do for yourself is to eat a protein-rich meal first thing in the morning. While you're sleeping, your body is using up its reserved energy, and you need to replenish it as soon as you can. The energy you give your body from breakfast is used up quickly, so it's a good idea to have an early lunch or at least have a nourishing snack a few hours after breakfast.

It's important that all meals contain protein, fat, and vegetable-based carbohydrates. (Avoiding simple carbohydrates is a must throughout the day.) You need all three components to fuel your body. Eating organic foods is your best choice. If you cannot afford to buy all organic, it is highly recommended that you eat organic meats and dairy products. There are many preservatives, hormones, and antibiotics added to nonorganic meat. Eating six to eight servings of vegetables a day is also recommended; eat as wide a variety of them as you can.

Digestive Problems

Opioid receptors found in the brain, spinal cord, and gastrointestinal tract are known to play a role in the function of the large intestines and gut in general.[164] Narcotic bowel syndrome (NBS) is a term that has been coined to describe narcotic-related digestive symptoms that resemble irritable bowel syndrome (IBS). NBS is not easily treated through Western medicine; while the "function" of digestion is obviously disrupted, there is no structural damage that can be found through testing.

While herbal therapy to resolve digestive issues can take many months, it does address the underlying causes, thus providing lasting relief. Acupuncture typically results in more immediate relief from digestive disorders.

TCM can address digestive issues such as IBS or NBS any number of ways depending on how the symptoms and the resulting imbalance present themselves. Let's look at two common patterns associated with digestive disorders in recovering opioid users.

Severe Liver Qi Stagnation

A common cause of digestive issues is Liver qi stagnation that has progressed and become severe; the condition is sometimes referred to as the "Liver attacking, or overacting on, the Large Intestine." This type of digestive disruption would likely become more active with emotional stress. Liver qi stagnation is seen in patterns with pain just below the ribs, agitation, insomnia between 1:00 and 3:00 a.m., premenstrual syndrome (PMS) or hormonal imbalances; see page 149 for more information.

Spleen Qi Deficiency and Digestion

The Spleen is one of the primary organ systems involved in digestion. Spleen qi deficiency is often associated with a poor diet that may include fried foods, sweets, refined foods, and an overconsumption of raw foods and iced drinks. Overthinking and worrying can also damage the Spleen function. Often, digestive problems related to Spleen qi deficiency will have elements of dampness, including sticky stools. Also, abdominal pain relieved with pressure or warmth to the area is common when there is Spleen qi deficiency (see Spleen organ system, page 34).

Constipation

One of the more common side effects of opioid use is constipation.[165] Simply discontinuing opioid use does not always result in the digestive system bouncing right back to full function. Herbal therapy and acupuncture, along with a diet rich in whole foods, can help to restore proper bowel movements.

SELF-TREATMENT OPTIONS FOR CONSTIPATION

- SINGLE HERBS: dandelion (page 83), yellow dock (page 97)

- ACUPRESSURE POINTS: ST 36 (page 65), LI 4 (page 66)

- ESSENTIAL OILS: dilute essential oils of coriander, fennel, and tangerine in olive oil (10% essential oils, 90% olive oil) and massage on the lower abdomen in large strokes in a clockwise motion

---

OPIOID-INDUCED CONSTIPATION RELIEF

While there are certainly herbs that quickly relieve constipation, such as cascara sagrada and senna leaf, these simply stimulate peristalsis of the intestines, and one can become dependent on them. Opioid-induced constipation is complex and requires a reset of the function of the large intestine and digestive system. This formula supports the entire process of elimination, beginning with stimulation of the gallbladder to release bile through bitter herbs. It is appropriate to use following withdrawal, rather than during it, and may take several months of use to provide long-term relief. For dosages, follow the recommendation of your licensed practitioner.

CHINESE NAME	ENGLISH NAME	PERCENTAGE OF FORMULA
Hu ma ren	Sesame seeds (black)	18.2%
Shan zha	Crataegus	13.9%
Mai ya	Barley sprouts (dry-fried)	13.6%
Lai fu zi	Raphanus	12.8%
Cang zhu	Atractylodes	10.3%
Gou qi zi	Lycium fruit	7.7%
Dang gui	Dong gui	4.8%
Pu gong ying	Dandelion	4.4%
Hu lu ba	Fenugreek seed	4.0%
Chen pi (ju pi)	Citrus peel (mature)	3.7%
Zhi shi	Citrus peel (green)	2.6%
Gan jiang	Ginger (dried)	2.2%
Long dan cao	Gentiana	1.8%

Heart Damage

It is well established that opioids have a strong negative impact on the heart.[166] What type of heart damage an opioid user might sustain will depend on three factors:

- Strength of dosing

- Length of use

- Personal constitution

TCM effectively treats heart disorders using acupuncture and herbs. See the discussion of the Heart organ system (page 33) for details.

High Blood Pressure

High blood pressure is a common malady seen in those who have been using or abusing opioids over a long time. Heart-Liver imbalance is typically implicated by high blood pressure; high blood pressure is an indication of Liver qi stagnation and Liver heat rising. You can address these issues by tonifying the Liver organ system (see the discussion on page 149).

Sleep Issues

Studies have shown that opioid use is associated with poor sleep quality; in one study, for example, people who reported using opioids were also 42 percent more likely to sleep poorly. Those taking high doses of opioids spend only 12.5 percent of their sleeping time in the deep rapid-eye movement (REM) sleep state, compared to 45 percent for people not taking opioids. Pain can also contribute to sleep disturbance, but poor sleep can be attributed to the disruptive brain changes that occur with opioid use.[167]

According to TCM, sleep disturbances are due to imbalances at the organ level, which must be corrected before sound sleep is restored. This explains why poor sleep continues after opioid use cessation. The Heart plays a central role in emotional disorders and sleep pattern problems. The Heart is said to "house the mind" during sleep.

Typically, trouble falling asleep points to a Heart qi deficiency or Heart shen disorder. Often, herbs that nourish the Heart shen (calming nervine herbs) are able to help people get to sleep.

There are several patterns that can be related to problems staying asleep, but the most common reason people wake through the night is blood and yin deficiency in the Heart. Blood is a dense substance that helps to ground the mind, and blood is a yin substance; without sufficient blood, the Heart is unable to contain, or ground, the mind at night. Those who suffer with more severe Heart blood deficiency may often find themselves waking startled and frightened. Someone who is blood deficient is not necessarily anemic; it simply indicates that there is not enough enriched blood to nourish all of the organs properly. This pattern may also include palpitations, a racing heart, or a sensation of the heart.

Dreams are normal, but having dreams so active that you wake unrested indicates an imbalance typically due to Heart heat. This can be produced from Liver qi stagnation causing Liver fire to rise, often consuming Heart blood and yin. Frightening dreams are often attributed to an imbalance of the Wood element and the Heart. With this type of insomnia, there may also be signs of Liver qi stagnation such as stress, frustration, anger, premenstrual syndrome (PMS), acid reflux, arthritis, or lack of motivation. Acid reflux in itself can often disturb sleep patterns. Many people fall into a pattern of waking between the hours of 1:00 and 3:00 a.m., almost like clockwork. This is typically an indication of Liver qi stagnation.

For treatment options, see the Calm Mind formula (page 176), as well as the general recommendations for Liver qi stagnation (page 149) and Kidney yin deficiency (page 142).

Immune Stress

Recovering opioid users often suffer from immune system deficiencies. As one 2016 article noted, "The effect of opioids on the immune system might be able to alter a variety of human body responses involving immune system, such as the response to stress, infection and malignant transformations [cancer]."[168] Exogenous and endogenous opioids both interact with the adaptive immune systems through the adrenal axis and the autonomic nervous system, as well as through opioid receptors located on immune cells. But while endogenous opioids benefit the body through immunoactivation, exogenous opioids from drug use have been shown to cause harm by causing immunosuppression.

According to TCM, *wei qi* (defensive energy; pronounced "way chee") circulates on the surface of the body, protecting the body from pathogens such as bacteria and viruses; this concept is loosely related to how modern medicine views the immune system. From the Chinese perspective, pathogens are ever present but do not generally pose a threat to health unless wei qi is weak and cannot protect the body.

TCM theory also dictates that when the body's resources are depleted, wei qi and qi in general are weakened and disease is more likely to take hold. Factors that deplete resources and weaken wei qi include unhealthy diet, inadequate sleep, and excessive amounts of damp weather or wind. As we've discussed, opioid dependency can effectively wipe out the body's resources, resulting in a lowered immune response. This weakened immune response can persist long after withdrawal if it is not addressed.

SELF-TREATMENT OPTIONS FOR IMMUNE STRESS

- SINGLE HERBS: astragalus (page 80), eleuthero (page 85), reishi (page 92)

- ESSENTIAL OILS: Nearly all essential oils benefit the immune system and are typically antibacterial and antiviral; try cypress (page 106), frankincense (page 107), or marjoram (page 112)

- ACUPRESSURE POINT: ST 36 (page 65)

This formula helps to restore immune health and wei qi through tonic and adaptogenic herbs. It is appropriate for those wanting to reestablish wellness after a long period of opioid use or abuse who are noticing a lowered immune response such as frequent colds and flus or autoimmune disorders. For dosages, follow the recommendation of your licensed practitioner.

CHINESE NAME	ENGLISH NAME	PERCENTAGE OF FORMULA
Wu jia pi	*Acanthopanax giraldii*	20.7%
Jiao gu lan	Gynostemma	18.0%
Huang qi (bei)	Astragalus root	13.4%
Wu wei zi	Schisandra	10.3%
Hong jing tian	Rhodiola	9.8%
Ling zhi (red)	Ganoderma (red)	8.2%
Bai zhu	Atractylodes (alba)	7.7%
Dang shen	Codonopsis	7.2%
Da zao (hong)	Jujube dates (red)	2.6%
Chen pi (ju pi)	Citrus peel (mature)	2.1%

Stress

One researcher has stated it clearly: "Stress is a well-known risk factor in the development of addiction and in addiction relapse vulnerability."[169] All of us have stressors in our lives; it is how we react to that stress that determines whether stress is going to negatively impact our health or behaviors. One person may be able to go with the flow during major life changes, while another person faced with the same situation may resort to drugs to mask stress and the resulting emotional imbalances that result.

It is known that our nervous system has two functional modes: the sympathetic and parasympathetic. To preserve adrenal health, we should live in the parasympathetic mode, which promotes a "rest and digest" response and a calming of the nerves.

Unfortunately, many of us are caught up in an unhealthy loop of emotional responses to life's everyday stresses, putting us in the sympathetic mode, which promotes a "fight or flight" response inhibiting digestion, increasing the heart rate, constricting blood vessels, inhibiting reproduction responses, and causing our body to consume tissue for quick energy.

TCM uses acupuncture, meditation, and adaptogenic herbs (see page 69) to rewire our brains so that we do not overreact to everyday stressors. These treatment modalities can especially be of benefit during withdrawal and recovery from opioid use, when patients can struggle to regain their equilibrium and normalize their stress response.

LIFESTYLE PRACTICES TO REDUCE STRESS RESPONSE

- Meditation for 15 to 30 minutes per day

- ½-mile walk three or four times per week

- Qi gong, tai chi, and/or yoga several times per week

Skin Issues

The health of the skin reflects the health of the body. People recovering from opioid dependency often suffer from poor health, and their skin can show it, with a sallow cast, dry patches, and slow healing of cuts and sores.

A classic symptom of opioid withdrawal is itchiness. According to TCM, this is less a skin issue than a result of internal wind that originates from Liver qi stagnation and resulting wind. See page 149 for treatment strategies.

As discussed earlier, opioid dependency is a stressor for the body and often coincides with nutritional imbalances, both of which contribute to skin issues. Another factor is the opioid toxins that accumulate in the body. Of course, the body deals with toxins every day from cleaning products, personal care products, and even the air we breathe. In most cases, the body can filter and eliminate toxins through natural avenues of elimination, one of which is the skin. However, when our health is compromised and our body is overloaded, these toxins can accumulate and ultimately damage the skin. In this situation, detoxification strategies can be helpful (see page 178).

Yin Deficiency and Dry Skin

Life stressors consume yin; opioid dependency does the same. Yin has moistening qualities, and its depletion can be reflected as dryness in the body and of the skin. Additionally, blood is a yin substance and is vital in its role in nourishing the skin. The beautiful rosy skin we enjoy throughout our youth can be attributed to abundant blood circulating throughout our body. Blood is vital in delivering nutrients to the cells, a fact that is reflected in a vibrant complexion and beautiful hair. For treatment options, see page 142.

Excessive Sweating

Sweats are common during the stress of withdrawal. However, many people who have long since stopped opioid use continue to experience abnormal episodes of sweating. These can be caused by one or more imbalances in the body.

Qi Deficiency and Sweating

Qi is responsible for holding the pores closed. One of the main indications of qi deficiency is sweating with no activity. Often, the resulting sweat feels greasier than normal sweat from activity. Other qi deficiency indications may also be present, such as loose stools, but sweating with no exertion is often an early indication of qi deficiency and can be seen alone. Qi deficiency is a common malady seen in opioid use because of poor nutritional habits. For treatment options, see the discussion of Spleen qi deficiency on page 160.

Kidney Yin Deficiency and Sweating

Common indications of yin deficiency are afternoon or night sweats; however, sweating from yin deficiency can occur at any time of the day or night. While often associated with menopausal women, yin deficiency can occur in women or men, and is common following extended opioid use. Yin represents substance in the body, and one of the main substances in our body is blood. Blood contains mostly water. Water, therefore blood, has an incredible insulative effect on the body, helping to moderate temperatures keep it warm when it is cold, and helping to keep it cool when it is warm. Some people think that simply drinking water will correct this problem; while it is true that hydrating is important, only yin foods and yin herbal tonics will reverse yin deficiency once it has developed in most cases. For treatment options, see the discussion of Kidney yin deficiency on page 142.

Notes

1. Center for Behavioral Health Statistics and Quality, *Results from the 2014 National Survey on Drug Use and Health: Detailed Tables* (Rockville, MD: Substance Abuse and Mental Health Services Administration, 2015), http://www.samhsa.gov/data/sites/default/files/NSDUH-DetTabs2014/NSDUH-DetTabs2014.pdf; Aaron D. Fox et al., "Release from Incarceration, Relapse to Opioid Use and the Potential for Buprenorphine Maintenance Treatment: A Qualitative Study of the Perceptions of Former Inmates with Opioid Use Disorder," *Addiction Science & Clinical Practice* 10, no. 2 (2015): 1–9; B. P. Smyth, J. Barry, E. Keenan, and K. Ducray, "Lapse and Relapse following Inpatient Treatment of Opiate Dependence," *Irish Medical Journal* 103, no. 6 (2010): 176–79; and National Institute on Drug Abuse, "America's Addiction to Opioids: Heroin and Prescription Drug Abuse," a presentation by Nora D. Volkow, M.D., to the U.S. Senate Caucus on International Narcotics Control, May 14, 2014, https://www.drugabuse.gov/about-nida/legislative-activities/testimony-to-congress/2016/americas-addiction-to-opioids-heroin-prescription-drug-abuse.

2. Arthur Yin Fan et al., "Acupuncture's Role in Solving the Opioid Epidemic: Evidence, Cost-Effectiveness, and Care Availability for Acupuncture as a Primary, Non-pharmacologic Method for Pain Relief and Management," *Journal of Integrative Medicine* 15, no. 6 (2017): 411–25.

3. Xueqi Wang et al., "Electroacupuncture Suppresses Morphine Reward-Seeking Behavior: Lateral Hypothalamic Orexin Neurons Implicated," *Neuroscience Letter* 661 (November 2017): 84–89.

4. Kenneth D. Kochanek et al., "Mortality in the United States, 2016," National Center for Health Statistics Data Brief no. 293 (December 2017).

5. Substance Abuse and Mental Health Services Administration, *Key Substance Use and Mental Health Indicators in the United States: Results from the 2016 National Survey on Drug Use and Health*, HHS publication no. SMA 17-5044, NSDUH series H-52 (Rockville, MD: Center for Behavioral Health Statistics and Quality, Substance Abuse and Mental Health Services Administration, 2017). https://www.samhsa.gov/data/.

6. Blue Cross Blue Shield website, https://www.bcbs.com, accessed June 2017.

7. Josh Katz, "Drug Deaths in America Are Rising Faster Than Ever," *New York Times*, June 5, 2017, https://www.nytimes.com/interactive/2017/06/05/upshot/opioid-epidemic-drug-overdose-deaths-are-rising-faster-than-ever.html, accessed June 2017.

8. Christopher Moraff, "Feds' Pill Crackdown Drives Pain Patients to Heroin," *Daily Beast*, April 15, 2016, https://www.thedailybeast.com/feds-pill-crackdown-drives-pain-patients-to-heroin, accessed June 2017.

9. Surgeon General, U.S. Department of Health and Human Services, "Surgeon General's Advisory on Nalaxone and

Opioid Drugs," April 5, 2018, https://www.surgeongeneral.gov/priorities/opioid-overdose-prevention/naloxone-advisory.html.

10. Jaymin Upadhyay et al., "Alterations in Brain Structure and Functional Connectivity in Prescription Opioid-Dependent Patients," *Brain* 133, no. 7 (2010): 2098–114; and Howard S. Smith, "Opioid Metabolism," *Mayo Clinic Proceedings* 84, no. 7 (2009): 613–24.

11. Upadhyay et al., "Alterations in Brain Structure."

12. Brown University, "Morphine Makes Lasting — and Surprising — Change in the Brain," *ScienceDaily*, April 26, 2007, https://www.sciencedaily.com/releases/2007/04/070425142116.htm.

13. Thomas R. Kosten and Tony P. George, "The Neurobiology of Opioid Dependence: Implications for Treatment," *Science & Practice Perspectives* 1, no. 1 (2002): 13–20.

14. Alvaro Pascual-Leone et al., "The Plastic Human Brain Cortex," *Annual Review of Neuroscience* 28 (2005): 377–401.

15. Jennifer C. Tomaszczyk et al., "Negative Neuroplasticity in Chronic Traumatic Brain Injury and Implications for Neurorehabilitation," *Neuropsychology Review* 24, no. 4 (2014): 409–27.

16. G. G. Xing et al., "Long-Term Synaptic Plasticity in the Spinal Dorsal Horn and Its Modulation by Electroacupuncture in Rats with Neuropathic Pain," *Experimental Neurology* 208, no. 2 (2007): 323–32; Vitaly Napadow et al., "Somatosensory Cortical Plasticity in Carpal Tunnel Syndrome — A Cross-Sectional Fmri Evaluation," *NeuroImage* 31, no. 2 (2006): 520–30; Vitaly Napadow et al., "Somatosensory Cortical Plasticity in Carpal Tunnel Syndrome Treated by Acupuncture," *Human Brain Mapping* 28, no. 3 (2007): 159–71; and Chun-Zhi Liu, Jian Kong, and KeLun Wang, "Acupuncture Therapies and Neuroplasticity," *Neural Plasticity* 2017 (April 27, 2017): Article ID 6178505.

17. Michael T. Treadway and Sara W. Lazar, "Meditation and Neuroplasticity: Using Mindfulness to Change the Brain," chapter 7 in *Assessing Mindfulness and Acceptance Processes in Clients,* ed. Ruth A. Baer (Oakland, CA: New Harbinger, 2010); and Richard J. Davidson and Antoine Lutz, "Buddha's Brain: Neuroplasticity and Meditation," *IEEE Signal Processing Magazine* 25, no. 1 (2008): 171–74.

18. AnGee Baldini, Michael Von Korff, and Elizabeth H. B. Lin, "A Review of Potential Adverse Effects of Long-Term Opioid Therapy: A Practitioner's Guide," *Primary Care Companion to CNS Disorders* 14, no. 3 (2012): PCC.11m01326; and National Institute on Drug Abuse, "Health Consequences of Drug Misuse," March 23, 2017, https://www.drugabuse.gov/related-topics/health-consequences-drug-misuse.

19. Jie Shi et al., "Traditional Chinese Medicine in Treatment of Opiate Addiction," *Acta Pharmacologica Sinica* 27, no. 10 (2006): 1303–8.

20. R. A. Deyo, M. Von Korff, and D. Duhrkoop, "Opioids for Low Back Pain," *BMJ* 350 (2015): g6380. doi:10.1136/bmj.g6380.

21. Icro Maremmani et al., "Subtyping Patients with Heroin Addiction at Treatment Entry: Factor Derived from the Self-Report Symptom Inventory (SCL-90)," *Annals of General Psychiatry* 9 (2010): 15.

22. Yuan Yu Chan et al., "The Benefit of Combined Acupuncture and Antidepressant Medication for Depression: A Systematic Review and Meta-analysis," *Journal of Affective Disorders* 176 (May 1, 2015): 106–17; and "Mandated Benefit Review of H.B. 3972: An Act Relative to the Practice of Acupuncture," Center for Health Information and Analysis, April 2015, http://www.aomsm .org/Resources/Documents/Research /BenefitReview-H3972-Acupuncture.pdf.

23. "New and Revised Standards Related to Pain Assessment and Management," *Joint Commission Perspectives* 37, no. 7 (July 2017): 3–4, https://www.jointcommission.org /assets/1/18/Joint_Commission_Enhances _Pain_Assessment_and_Management _Requirements_for_Accredited_Hospitals1 .PDF.

24. K. Beltaief et al., "Acupuncture versus Titrated Morphine in Acute Renal Colic: A Randomized Controlled Trial," *Journal of Pain Research* 11 (2018): 335–41. doi:10.2147 /JPR.S136299.

25. Dario Tedesco et al., "Drug-Free Interventions to Reduce Pain or Opioid Consumption after Total Knee Arthroplasty: A Systematic Review and Meta-analysis," *JAMA Surgery* 152, no. 10 (2017): e172872; Shun Huang et al., "Effects of Transcutaneous Electrical Acupoint Stimulation at Different Frequencies on Perioperative Anesthetic Dosage, Recovery, Complications, and Prognosis in Video-Assisted Thoracic Surgical Lobectomy: A Randomized, Double-Blinded, Placebo-Controlled Trial," *Journal of Anesthesia.* 31, no. 1 (2017): 58–65; Sven Asmussen et al., "Meta-Analysis of Electroacupuncture in Cardiac Anesthesia and Intensive Care," *Journal of Intensive Care Medicine* (2017); Li-Xin An et al., "Electro-Acupuncture Decreases Postoperative Pain and Improves Recovery in Patients Undergoing a Supratentorial Craniotomy," *American Journal of Chinese Medicine* 42, no. 5 (2014): 1099–1109; and Sven Asmussen et al., "Effects of Acupuncture in Anesthesia for Craniotomy: A Meta-Analysis," *Journal of Neurosurgical Anesthesiology* 29, no. 3 (2017): 219–27.

26. Juang-Geng Lin et al., "The Effect of High and Low Frequency Electroacupuncture in Pain after Lower Abdominal Surgery," *Pain* 99, no. 3 (2002): 509–14; and Baoguo Wang et al., "Effect of the Intensity of Transcutaneous Acupoint Electrical Stimulation on the Postoperative Analgesic Requirement," *Anesthesia and Analgesia* 85, no. 2 (1997): 406–13.

27. U.S. Centers for Disease Control and Prevention, National Center for Health Statistics, FastStats, "Ambulatory Care Use and Physician Office Visits," https://www .cdc.gov/nchs/fastats/physician-visits.htm, accessed March 31, 2018.

28. R. Chou et al., "Nonpharmacologic Therapies for Low Back Pain: A Systematic Review for an American College of Physicians Clinical Practice Guideline," *Annals of Internal Medicine* 166, no. 7 (2017): 493–505; and Amir Qaseem et al., "Noninvasive Treatments for Acute, Subacute, and Chronic Low Back Pain: A Clinical Practice Guideline from the American College of Physicians," *Annals of Internal Medicine* 166, no. 7 (2017): 514–30.

29. Paul Crawford, Donald B. Penzien, and Remy Coeytaux, "Reduction in Pain Medication Prescriptions and Self-Reported Outcomes Associated with Acupuncture in a Military Patient Population," *Medical Acupuncture* 29, no. 4 (2017): 229–31.

30. Benjamin Kligler, "Integrative Health in the Veterans Health Administration," *Medical Acupuncture* 29, no. 4 (August 2017): 187–88; and Joseph M. Helms, "Medical Acupuncture Meets the Military," *Medical Acupuncture* 29, no. 4 (2017): 189–90.

31. M. S. Corbett et al., "Acupuncture and other Physical Treatments for the Relief of Pain Due to Osteoarthritis of the Knee: Network Meta-analysis," *Osteoarthritis and Cartilage* 21, no. 9 (2013): 1290–98; John McDonald and Stephen Janz, *The Acupuncture Evidence Project: A Comprehensive Literature Review*, rev. ed. (Brisbane: Australian Acupuncture & Chinese Medicine Association Limited, 2017); Andrew J. Vickers et al., "Acupuncture for Chronic Pain: Individual Patient Data Meta-Analysis," *Archives of Internal Medicine* 172, no. 19 (2012): 1444–53; and Marcus Gadau et al., "Acupuncture and Moxibustion for Lateral Elbow Pain: A Systematic Review of Randomized Controlled Trials," *BMC Complementary and Alternative Medicine* 14 (2014): 136.

32. "Mandated Benefit Review of H.B. 3972: An Act Relative to the Practice of Acupuncture," Center for Health Information and Analysis, April 2015, http://www.aomsm .org/Resources/Documents/Research /BenefitReview-H3972-Acupuncture.pdf.

33. F. E. Motlagh, F. Ibrahim, R. A. Rashid, T. Seghatoleslam, and H. Habil, "Acupuncture Therapy for Drug Addiction," *Chinese Medicine* 11, no. 16 (2017). doi:10.1186 /s13020-016-0088-7.

34. Jaung-Geng Lin, Yuan-Yu Chan, and Yi-Hung Chen, "Acupuncture for the Treatment of Opiate Addiction," *Evidence-Based Complementary and Alternative Medicine* 2012 (2012). doi:10.1155/2012/739045.

35. Liu-Zhen Wu et al., "Suppression of Morphine Withdrawal by Electroacupuncture in Rats: Dynorphin and Kappa-Opioid Receptor Implicated," *Brain Research* 851, nos. 1–2 (1999): 290–96.

36. Bei-Hung Chang and Elizabeth Sommers, "Acupuncture and Relaxation Response for Craving and Anxiety Reduction among Military Veterans in Recovery from Substance Use Disorder," *American Journal of Addiction* 23, no. 2 (2014): 129–36.

37. National Acupuncture Detoxification Association, "About NADA," http://www .acudetox.com/about-nada/12faqs2013.

38. Diane Swengros et al., "Promoting Caring-Healing Relationships: Bringing Healing Touch to the Bedside in a Multihospital Health System," *Holistic Nurse Practitioner* 28, no. 6 (2014): 370–75; and Joel G. Anderson et al., "The Effects of Healing Touch on Pain, Nausea, and Anxiety Following Bariatric Surgery: A Pilot Study," *Explore* 11, no. 3 (2015): 208–16.

39. J. W. Boland, G. A. Foulds, S. H. Ahmedzai, and A. G. Pockley, "A Preliminary Evaluation of the Effects of Opioids on Innate and Adaptive Human In Vitro Immune Function," *BMJ Supportive and Palliative Care* 4, no. 4 (2014): 357–67.

40. B. Pajusco et al., "Tobacco Addiction and Smoking Status in Heroin Addicts under Methadone vs. Buprenorphine Therapy," *International Journal of Environmental Research and Public Health* 9, no. 3 (2012): 932–42. doi:10.3390 /ijerph9030932.

41. U.S. National Institutes of Health, LiverTox, "Drug Record: Opioids, Opioid Antagonists," https://livertox.nlm.nih.gov/Opioids .htm#overview, accessed March 31, 2018.

42. H. Hedegaard, M. Warner, and A. Minino, "Drug Overdose Deaths in the United States, 1999–2016," U.S. Centers for Disease Control and Prevention, National Center for Health Statistics, NCHS Data Brief no. 294 (December 2017), https://www.cdc.gov/nchs/products/databriefs/db294.htm.

43. Ian Musgrave, "Study Reveals That Nearly 90% of Traditional Chinese Medicines Contain Trace Amounts of Disturbing and Toxic Substances," Business Insider, December 13, 2015, http://www.businessinsider.com/study-reveals-chinese-medicines-contain-trace-amounts-of-toxic-substances-2015-12.

44. Morgan A. Pratte et al., "An Alternative Treatment for Anxiety: A Systematic Review of Human Trial Results Reported for the Ayurvedic Herb Ashwagandha (*Withania somnifera*)," *Journal of Alternative and Complementary Medicine* 20, no. 12 (December 2014): 901–8.

45. Manuel Candelario et al., "Direct Evidence for GABAergic Activity of *Withania somnifera* on Mammalian Ionotropic GABAA and GABAρ Receptors," *Journal of Ethnopharmacology* 171 (August 2, 2015): 264–72.

46. Dnyanraj Choudhary, Sauvik Bhattacharyya, and Kedar Joshi et al., "Body Weight Management in Adults under Chronic Stress through Treatment with Ashwagandha Root Extract: A Double-Blind, Randomized, Placebo-Controlled Trial," *Journal of Evidence-Based Complementary Inegrative Medicine* 22, no. 1 (January 2017): 96–106.

47. Yue Wang et al., "*Astragalus saponins* Inhibits Lipopolysaccharide-Induced Inflammation in Mouse Macrophages," *American Journal of Chinese Medicine* 44,

no. 3 (2016): 579–93; Kathy K. Auyeung, Quin-Ban Han, and Joshua K. Ko, "*Astragalus membranaceus*: A Review of Its Protection against Inflammation and Gastrointestinal Cancers," *American Journal of Chinese Medicine* 44, no. 1 (2016): 1–22; and Wei Wei et al., "TLR-4 May Mediate Signaling Pathways of *Astragalus* Polysaccharide RAP Induced Cytokine Expression of RAW264.7 Cells," *Journal of Ethnopharmacology* 179 (2016): 243–52.

48. Chien-Liang Chao et al., "Sesquiterpenes from Baizhu Stimulate Glucose Uptake by Activating AMPK and PI3K," *American Journal of Chinese Medicine* 44, no. 5 (2016): 963–79.

49. Fangyi Long et al., "Anti-Tumor Effects of Atractylenolide-I on Human Ovarian Cancer Cells," *Medical Science Monitor* 23 (2017): 571–79.

50. Na Zhang et al., "Two New Compounds from *Atractylodes macrocephala* with Neuroprotective Activity," *Journal of Asian Natural Products Research* 19, no. 1 (January 2017): 35–41; and Xin Fu et al., "New Hope for Alzheimer's Disease," *Aging and Disease* 7, no. 4 (August 2016): 502–13.

51. Le Son Hoang et al., "Inflammatory Inhibitory Activity of Sesquiterpenoids from *Atractylodes macrocephala* Rhizomes," *Chemical and Pharmceutical Bulletin* 64, no. 5 (2016): 507–11.

52. Suresh Awale et al., "Identification of Arctigenin as an Antitumor Agent Having the Ability to Eliminate the Tolerance of Cancer Cells to Nutrient Starvation," *Cancer Research* 66, no. 3 (2006): 1751–57; and Siti Susanti et al., "Tumor Specific Cytotoxicity of Arctigenin Isolated from Herbal Plant

Arctium lappa L.," *Journal of Natural Medicines* 66, no. 4 (2012): 614–21.

53. Song-Chow Lin et al., "Hepatoprotective Effects of *Arctium lappa* Linne on Liver Injuries Induced by Chronic Ethanol Consumption and Potentiated by Carbon Tetrachloride," *Journal of Biomedical Science* 9, no. 5 (2002): 401–9.

54. Akram Ahangarpour et al., "Antidiabetic, Hypolipidemic and Hepatoprotective Effects of *Arctium lappa* Root's Hydro-alcoholic Extract on Nicotinamide-Streptozotocin Induced Type 2 Model of Diabetes in Male Mice," *Avicenna Journal of Phytomedicine* 7, no. 2 (2017): 169–79.

55. National Academies of Sciences, Engineering, and Medicine, *The Health Effects of Cannabis and Cannabinoids: The Current State of Evidence and Recommendations for Research* (Washington, DC: The National Academies Press, 2017).

56. Philippe Lucas, "Rationale for Cannabis-Based Interventions in the Opioid Overdose Crisis," *Harm Reduction Journal* 14, no. 58 (2017).

57. Kevin F. Boehnke, Evangelos Litinas, and Daniel J. Clauw, "Medical Cannabis Use Is Associated with Decreased Opiate Medication Use in a Retrospective Cross-Sectional Survey of Patients with Chronic Pain," *Journal of Pain* 17, no. 6 (2016): 739–44.

58. National Academies of Sciences, *Health Effects of Cannabis.*

59. Yong-Xu Sun, "Immunological Adjuvant Effect of a Water-Soluble Polysaccharide, CPP, from the Roots of *Codonopsis pilosula*

on the Immune Responses to Ovalbumin in Mice," *Chemistry & Biodiversity* 6, no. 6 (June 2009): 890–96.

60. Chong Xu et al., "The Contribution of Side Chains to Antitumor Activity of a Polysaccharide from *Codonopsis pilosula*," *International Journal of Biological Macromolecules* 50, no. 4 (May 1, 2012): 891–94; and Xu Chu et al., "Effects of *Astragalus* and *Codonopsis pilosula* Polysaccharides on Alveolar Macrophage Phagocytosis and Inflammation in Chronic Obstructive Pulmonary Disease Mice Exposed to PM2.5," *Environmental Toxicology and Pharmacology* 48 (December 2016): 76–84.

61. Dirleise Colle et al., "Antioxidant Properties of *Taraxacum officinale* Leaf Extract Are Involved in the Protective Effect against Hepatoxicity Induced by Acetaminophen in Mice," *Journal of Medicinal Food* 15, no. 6 (2012): 549–56; and Muhammad Gulfraz et al., "Effect of Leaf Extracts of *Taraxacum officinale* on CCl4 Induced Hepatotoxicity in Rats, *In Vivo* Study," *Pakistan Journal of Pharmaceutical Science* 27, no. 4 (2014): 825–29.

62. Munkhtugs Davaatseren et al., "*Taraxacum official* (Dandelion) Leaf Extract Alleviates High-Fat Diet-Induced Nonalcoholic Fatty Liver," *Food and Chemical Toxicology* 58 (August 2013): 30–36.

63. Jing Wang et al., "Isoalantolactone Inhibits the Migration and Invasion of Human Breast Cancer MDA-MB-231 Cells via Suppression of the p38 MAPK/NF-κB Signaling Pathway," *Oncololgy Reports* 36, no. 3 (2016): 1269–76.

64. Shuang Gao et al., "Total Sesquiterpene Lactones Prepared from *Inula helenium* L. Has Potentials in Prevention and Therapy of Rheumatoid Arthritis," *Journal of Ethnopharmacolology* 196 (2017): 39–46.

65. Lin-Zhang Huang et al., "Antifatigue Activity of the Liposoluble Fraction from *Acanthopanax senticosus*," *Phytotherapy Research* 25, no. 6 (June 2011): 940–43.

66. Alexander Panossian et al., "Adaptogens Stimulate Neuropeptide Y and Hsp72 Expression and Release in Neuroglia Cells," *Frontiers in Neuroscience* 6, no. 6 (February 1, 2012).

67. Ji-Nian Fang, A. Proksch, and Hildebert Wagner, "Immunologically Active Polysaccharides of *Acanthopanax senticosus*," *Phytochemistry* 24, no. 11 (1985): 2619–22.

68. Sun Young Park et al., "Anti-inflammatory Effects of Novel Polygonum Multiflorum Compound via Inhibiting NF-κB/MAPK and Upregulating the Nrf2 Pathways in LPS-Stimulated Microglia," *Neuroscience Letters* 651 (June 9, 2017): 43–51; and Rui Li et al., "Antiaging and Anxiolytic Effects of Combinatory Formulas Based on Four Medicinal Herbs," *Evidence-Based Complementary and Alternative Medicine* 2017 (2017): Article ID 4624069.

69. Chunyu Li et al., "Screening for Main Components Associated with the Idiosyncratic Hepatotoxicity of a Tonic Herb, *Polygonum multiflorum*," *Frontiers of Medicine* 11, no. 2 (2017): 253–65.

70. Ya-Min Hou, Jie Wang, and Xian-Zhao Zhang, "Lycium Barbarum Polysaccharide Exhibits Cardioprotection in an Experimental Model of Ischemia-Reperfusion Damage," *Molecular Medicine Report* 15, no. 5 (2017): 2653–58; and You Jin Lee et al., "Dietary Wolfberry Extract Modifies Oxidative Stress by Controlling the Expression of Inflammatory mRNAs in Overweight and Hypercholesterolemic Subjects: A Randomized, Double-Blind, Placebo-Controlled Trial," *Journal of Agricultural Food Chemistry* 65, no. 2 (2017): 309–16.

71. Mi Hye Kim et al., "Improvement of Osteoporosis by Lycium Chinense Administration in Ovariectomized Mice," *Journal of the Chinese Medical Association* 80, no. 4 (2017): 222–26.

72. Ilkay Erdogan Orhan, "Phytochemical and Pharmacological Activity Profile of *Crataegus oxyacantha* L. (Hawthorn) — A Cardiotonic Herb," *Current Medical Chemistry* 23 (2016); Simone Fuchs et al., "The Dual Edema-Preventing Molecular Mechanism of the Crataegus Extract WS 1442 Can Be Assigned to Distinct Phytochemical Fractions," *Planta Medica* 83, no. 8 (2017): 701–9; Gary N. Asher et al., "Effect of Hawthorn Standardized Extract on Flow Mediated Dilation in Prehypertensive and Mildly Hypertensive Adults: A Randomized, Controlled Cross-over Trial," *BMC Complementary and Alternative Medicine* 12, no. 26 (2012); and Abdoulaye Diane et al., "Hypolipidemic and Cardioprotective Benefits of a Novel Fireberry Hawthorn Fruit Extract in the JCR:LA-cp Rodent Model of Dyslipidemia and Cardiac Dysfunction," *Food & Function* 7, no. 9 (2016): 3943–52.

73. Yantao Li et al., "Anti-cancer Effects of *Gynostemma pentaphyllum* (Thunb.) Makino (*Jiaogulan*)," *Chinese Medicine* 11, no. 43 (2016).

74. Ezarul Lokman et al., "Evaluation of Antidiabetic Effects of the Traditional Medicinal Plant *Gynostemma pentaphyllum*

and the Possible Mechanisms of Insulin Release," *Evidence-Based Complementary Alternative Medicine* 2015 (2015): Article ID 120572.

75. Qin He et al., "Mechanism of Action of Gypenosides on Type 2 Diabetes and Non-alcoholic Fatty Liver Disease in Rats," *World Journal of Gastroenterology* 21, no. 7 (2015): 2058–66.

76. Eduardo Cinosi et al., "Following 'the Roots' of Kratom (*Mitragyna speciosa*): The Evolution of an Enhancer from a Traditional Use to Increase Work and Productivity in Southeast Asia to a Recreational Psychoactive Drug in Western Countries," *BioMed Research International* (2015): Article ID 968786.

77. Batool Rahmati et al., "Antidepressant and Anxiolytic Activity of *Lavandula officinalis* Aerial Parts Hydroalcoholic Extract in Scopolamine-Treated Rats," *Pharmceutical Biology* 55, no. 1 (2017): 958–65.

78. Ji Hyun Baek, Andrew A. Nierenberg, and Gustavo Kinrys, "Clinical Applications of Herbal Medicines for Anxiety and Insomnia; Targeting Patients with Bipolar Disorder," *Australian & New Zealand Journal of Psychiatry* 48, no. 8 (2014): 705–15; and Abolfazl Shakeri, Amirhossein Sahebkar, and Behjat Javadi, "*Melissa officinalis* L. — A Review of Its Traditional Uses, Phytochemistry and Pharmacology," *Journal of Ethnopharmacology* 188 (2016): 204–28.

79. Daniil N. Olennikov, Nina I. Kashchenko, and Nadezhda K. Chirikova, "Meadowsweet Teas as New Functional Beverages: Comparative Analysis of Nutrients, Phytochemicals and Biological Effects of Four Filipendula Species," *Molecules* 22, no. 1 (2017): 16; Jelena Katanić et al., "*In Vitro* and *In Vivo* Assessment of Meadowsweet

(*Filipendula ulmaria*) as Anti-inflammatory Agent," *Journal of Ethnopharmacology* 193 (2016): 627–36; Anca Toiu et al., "HPLC Analysis of Salicylic Derivatives from Natural Products," *Farmacia* 59, no. 1 (2011): 106–12; and Jeanette Wick, "Aspirin: A History, a Love Story," *Consultant Pharmacist* 27, no. 5 (2012): 322–29.

80. Simon Mills and Kerry Bone, *Principles and Practice of Phytotherapy: Modern Herbal Medicine* (Edinburgh: Churchill Livingstone, 2000), 60–61, 148–49, 479–82.

81. Katarzyna Wojtyniak, Marcin Szymański, and Irena Matławska, "*Leonurus cardiaca* L. (Motherwort): A Review of Its Phytochemistry and Pharmacology," *Phytotherapy Research* 27, no. 8 (2013): 1115–20.

82. Alexander N. Shikov et al., "Effect of *Leonurus cardiaca* Oil Extract in Patients with Arterial Hypertension Accompanied by Anxiety and Sleep Disorders," *Phytotherapy Research* 25, no. 4 (2011): 540–43.

83. Kurt Appel et al., "Modulation of the γ-Aminobutyric Acid (GABA) System by *Passiflora incarnata* L.," *Phytotherapy Research* 25, no. 6 (June 2011): 838–43.

84. James Ahn et al., "Natural Product-Derived Treatments for Attention-Deficit/Hyperactivity Disorder: Safety, Efficacy, and Therapeutic Potential of Combination Therapy," *Neural Plasticity* (2016): Article ID 1320423.

85. Urooj Aman et al., "*Passiflora incarnata* Attenuation of Neuropathic Allodynia and Vulvodynia Apropos GABA-ergic and Opioidergic Antinociceptive and Behavioural Mechanisms," *BMC Complementary and Alternative Medicine* 16, no. 77 (2016).

86. Chun Hay Ko et al., "Multitargeted Combination Effects of a Tri-herbal Formulation Containing ELP against Osteoporosis: *In Vitro* Evidence," *Journal of Pharmacy and Pharmacology* 68, no. 6 (2016): 826–33.

87. Xiao-peng Hu et al., "Anti-influenza Virus Effects of Crude Phenylethanoid Glycosides Isolated from *Ligustrum purpurascens* via Inducing Endogenous Interferon-γ," *Journal of Ethnopharmacology* 179 (2016): 128–36; V. Katalinic et al., "Screening of 70 Medicinal Plant Extracts for Antioxidant Capacity and Total Phenols," *Food Chemistry* 94 (2006): 550–57; and Hye Lim Seo et al., "*Liqustri lucidi* Fructus Inhibits Hepatic Injury and Functions as an Antioxidant by Activation of AMP-Activated Protein Kinase *In Vivo* and *In Vitro*," *Chemico-Biological Interactions* 262 (2017): 57–68.

88. Cheng-Chieh Chang et al., "Oxidative Stress and *Salvia miltiorrhiza* in Aging-Associated Cardiovascular Diseases," *Oxidative Medicine and Cellular Longevity* 2016 (2016): Article ID 4797102.

89. Laura Bonaccini et al., "Effects of *Salvia miltiorrhiza* on CNS Neuronal Injury and Degeneration: A Plausible Complementary Role of Tanshinones and Depsides," *Planta Medica* 81, nos. 12–13 (2015): 1003–16; and Chun-Yan Su et al., "*Salvia miltiorrhiza*: Traditional Medicinal Uses, Chemistry, and Pharmacology," *Chinese Journal of Natural Medicines* 13, no. 3 (2015): 163–82.

90. Yuan Yuan et al., "Advance in Studies on Hepatoprotective Effect of *Salvia miltiorrhiza* and Its Main Components," *Zhongguo Zhong Yao Za Zhi* 40, no. 4 (2015): 588–93.

91. Antonnio Barbieri et al., "Anticancer and Anti-Inflammatory Properties of *Ganoderma lucidum* Extract Effects on Melanoma and Triple-Negative Breast Cancer Treatment," *Nutrients* 9, no. 3 (2017): 210; Balraj Singh Gill, Sanjeev Kumar, and Navgeet, "Ganoderic Acid Targeting Nuclear Factor Erythroid 2-Related Factor 2 in Lung Cancer," *Tumor Biology* 39, no. 3 (2017): 1–12; and Kun Na et al., "Anticarcinogenic Effects of Water Extract of Sporoderm-Broken Spores of *Ganoderma lucidum* on Colorectal Cancer *In Vitro* and *In Vivo*," *Internal Journal of Oncology* 50, no. 5 (2017): 1541–54.

92. Deng Pan et al., "Antidiabetic, Antihyperlipidemic and Antioxidant Activities of a Novel Proteoglycan from *Ganoderma lucidum* Fruiting Bodies on db/db Mice and the Possible Mechanism," *PLoS One* 8, no. 7 (2013): e68332.

93. Fangjiao Song et al., "Schizandrin A Inhibits Microglia-Mediated Neuroinflammation through Inhibiting TRAF6-NF-κB and Jak2-Stat3 Signaling Pathways," *PLoS One* 11, no. 2 (2016): e0149991.

94. Tingxu Yan et al., "Lignans from *Schisandra chinensis* Ameliorate Cognition Deficits and Attenuate Brain Oxidative Damage Induced by D-galactose in Rats," *Metabolic Brain Disease* 31, no. 3 (2016): 653–61.

95. K. M. Ko et al., "Effect of a Lignan-Enriched Fructus Schisandrae Extract on Hepatic Glutathione Status in Rats: Protection against Carbon Tetrachloride Toxicity," *Planta Medica* 61, no. 2 (1995): 134–37.

96. Shobhit Srivastava et al., "*Curcuma longa* Extract Reduces Inflammatory and Oxidative Stress Biomarkers in Osteoarthritis of Knee: A Four-Month, Double-Blind,

Randomized, Placebo-Controlled Trial," *Inflammopharmacology* 24, no. 6 (2016): 377–88; K. Madhu, Chanda Kulkarni, and M. J. Saji, "Safety and Efficacy of *Curcuma longa* Extract in the Treatment of Painful Knee Osteoarthritis: A Randomized Placebo-Controlled Trial," *Inflammopharmacology* 21, no. 2 (2013): 129–36; and Ashok Kumar Grover and Sue E. Samson, "Benefits of Antioxidant Supplements for Knee Osteoarthritis: Rationale and Reality," *Nutrition Journal* 15, no. 1 (2016).

97. H. Hatcher, et al., "Curcumin: From Ancient Medicine to Current Clinical Trials," *Cellular and Molecular Life Sciences*, 65, no. 11 (2008): 1631–52.

98. Feng-Mei Qiu et al., "The Antidepressant-Like Effects of Paeoniflorin in Mouse Models," *Experimental and Therapeutic Medicine* 5, no. 4 (2013): 1113–16; and Feng-Mei Qiu et al., "Antidepressant-like Effects of Paeoniflorin on the Behavioral, Biochemical, and Neurochemical Patterns of Rats Exposed to Chronic Unpredictable Stress," *Neuroscience Letters* 541 (2013): 209–13.

99. Zhenyu Zhou et al., "Paeoniflorin Prevents Hypoxia-Induced Epithelial-Mesenchymal Transition in Human Breast Cancer Cells," *Oncology Targets and Therapy* 2016, no. 9 (2016): 2511–18.

100. A. Wesołowska et al., "Analgesic and Sedative Activities of Lactucin and Some Lactucin-Like Guaianolides in Mice," *Journal of Ethnopharmacology* 107, no. 2 (2006): 254–58.

101. Ibid.

102. Sima Besharat, Mahsa Besharat, and Ali Jabbari, "Wild Lettuce (*Lactuca virosa*) Toxicity," *BMJ Case Reports* (2009). doi: 10.1136/bcr.06.2008.0134.

103. Ensiyeh Jenabi and Bita Fereidoony, "Effect of *Achillea millefolium* on Relief of Primary Dysmenorrhea: A Double-Blind Randomized Clinical Trial," *Journal of Pediatric & Adolescent Gynecology* 28, no. 5 (2015): 402–4; and Maryam Hajhashemi et al., "The Effect of *Achillea millefolium* and *Hypericum perforatum* Ointments on Episiotomy Wound Healing in Primiparous Women," *Journal of Maternal-Fetal & Neonatal Medicine* 31, no. 1 (2018): 63–69.

104. Zoran Maksimović et al., "Antioxidant Activity of Yellow Dock (*Rumex crispus* L., Polygonaceae) Fruit Extract," *Phytotherapy Research* 25, no. 1 (2011): 101–5; and Supriya Shiwani, Naresh Kumar Singh, and Myeong Hyeon Wang, "Carbohydrase Inhibition and Anti-cancerous and Free Radical Scavenging Properties along with DNA and Protein Protection Ability of Methanolic Root Extracts of *Rumex crispus*," *Nutrition Research and Practice* 6, no. 5 (2012): 389–95.

105. Xuesheng Han and Tory L. Parker, "Antiinflammatory Activity of Cinnamon (*Cinnamomum zeylanicum*) Bark Essential Oil in a Human Skin Disease Model," *Phytotherapy Research* 31, no. 7 (2017): 1034–38.

106. Xuesheng Han and Tory L. Parker, "Anti-inflammatory Activity of Clove (*Eugenia caryophyllata*) Essential Oil in Human Dermal Fibroblasts," *Pharmaceutical Biology* 55, no. 1 (2017): 1619–22.

107. M. A. Davis, L. A. Lin, H. Liu, and B. D. Sites, "Prescription Opioid Use among Adults with Mental Health Disorders in the United States," *Journal of the American Board of Family Medicine* 30, no. 4 (2017): 407–17.

108. E. Bach, *The Twelve Healers and Other Remedies* (Pilgrims Publishing, 2002), 25.

109. Ibid.

110. Sepideh Nabipour, Mas Ayu Said, and Mohd Hussain Habil, "Burden and Nutritional Deficiencies in Opioid Addiction — Systematic Review Article," *Iran Journal of Public Health* 43, no. 8 (2014): 1022–32.

111. Ibid.

112. Lawrence Feinman, "Absorption and Utilization of Nutrients in Alcoholism," *Alcohol Health & Research World* 13, no. 3 (1989): 207–10.

113. John Finnegan and Daphne Gray, *Recovery from Addiction: A Comprehensive Understanding of Substance Abuse with Nutritional Therapies for Recovering Addicts and Co-dependents* (Berkeley, CA: Celestial Arts, 1990); Mihai Nechifor, "Magnesium in Drug Dependences," *Magnesium Research* 21, no. 1 (2008): 5–15; and George A. Eby and Karen L. Eby, "Rapid Recovery from Major Depression Using Magnesium Treatment," *Medical Hypotheses* 67, no. 2 (2006): 362–70.

114. Malcolm Peet and Caroline Stokes, "Omega-3 Fatty Acids in the Treatment of Psychiatric Disorders," *Drugs* 65, no. 8 (2005): 1051–59.

115. Wojciech Leppert, "The Impact of Opioid Analgesics on the Gastrointestinal Tract Function and the Current Management Possibilities," *Contemporary Oncology* 16, no. 2 (2012): 125–31; and Tiziana Larussa, Maria Imeneo, and Francesco Luzza, "Potential Role of Nutraceutical Compounds in Inflammatory Bowel Disease," *World Journal of Gastroenterology* 14, no. 23 (2017): 2483–92.

116. John E. Lewis et al., "The Effect of Methylated Vitamin B Complex on Depressive and Anxiety Symptoms and Quality of Life in Adults with Depression," *International Scholarly Research Notes: Psychiatry* (2013): Article ID 621453.

117. Angela Sorice et al., "Ascorbic Acid: Its Role in Immune System and Chronic Inflammation Diseases," *Mini Reviews in Medicinal Chemisry* 14, no. 5 (2014): 444–52.

118. A. Evangelou et al., "Ascorbic Acid (Vitamin C) Effects on Withdrawal Syndrome of Heroin Abusers," *In Vivo* 14, no. 2 (2000): 363–66.

119. Kathleen DesMaisons, *Potatoes Not Prozac: A Natural Seven-Step Dietary Plan to Control Your Cravings and Lose Weight* (Old Tappan, NJ: Fireside 1999), 79.

120. Lukas Pezawas et al., "5-HTTLPR Polymorphism Impacts Human Cingulate-Amygdala Interactions: A Genetic Susceptibility Mechanism for Depression," *Nature Neuroscience* 8, no. 6 (2005): 828–34.

121. J. A. Schinka, R. M. Busch, and N. Robichaux-Keene, "A Meta-analysis of the Association between the Serotonin Transporter Gene Polymorphism (5-HTTLPR) and Trait Anxiety," *Molecular Psychiatry* 9, no. 2 (2004): 197–202.

122. Jessica M. Yano et al., "Indigenous Bacteria from the Gut Microbiota Regulate Host Serotonin Biosynthesis," *Cell* 161, no. 2 (2015): 264–76.

123. Andrzej Slominski et al., "Conversion of L-Tryptophan to Serotonin and Melatonin in Human Melanoma Cells," *FEBS Letters* 511, nos. 1–3 (2002): 102–6.

124. Adham M. Abdou et al., "Relaxation and Immunity Enhancement Effects of γ-Aminobutyric Acid (GABA)

Administration in Humans," *Biofactors* 26, no. 3 (2006): 201–8.

125. Laura Steenbergen et al., "Transcutaneous Vagus Nerve Stimulation (tVNS) Enhances Response Selection during Action Cascading Processes," *European Neuropsychopharmacology* 25, no. 6 (2015): 773–78.

126. Tsutomu Kanehira et al., "Relieving Occupational Fatigue by Consumption of a Beverage Containing γ-Amino Butyric Acid," *Journal of Nutritional Science and Vitaminology* 57, no. 1 (2011): 9–15.

127. Masahito Watanabe et al., "GABA and GABA Receptors in the Central Nervous System and Other Organs," *International Review of Cytology* 213 (2002): 1–47.

128. D. D. Rasmussen et al., "Effects of Tyrosine and Tryptophan Ingestion on Plasma Catecholamine and 3,4-Dihydroxyphenylacetic Acid Concentrations," *Journal of Clinical Endocrinology and Metabolism* 57, no. 4 (1983): 760–63.

129. Wolfram Schultz, "Neuronal Reward and Decision Signals: From Theories to Data," *Physiological Reviews* 95, no. 3 (2015): 853–951.

130. Eric J. Nestler, "Transcriptional Mechanisms of Drug Addiction," *Clinical Psychopharmacology and Neuroscience* 10, no. 3 (2012): 136–43.

131. Rajita Sinha, "The Clinical Neurobiology of Drug Craving," *Current Opinion in Neurobiology* 23, no. 4 (2013): 649–54; and B. T. Thomas Yeo et al., "The Organization of the Human Cerebral Cortex Estimated by Intrinsic Functional Connectivity," *Journal of Neurophysiology* 106, no. 3 (2011): 1125–65.

132. Harris R. Lieberman et al., "The Effects of Dietary Neurotransmitter Precursors on Human Behavior," *American Journal of Clinical Nutrition* 42, no. 2 (1985): 366–70; Richard A. Magill et al., "Effects of Tyrosine, Phentermine, Caffeine D-Amphetamine, and Placebo on Cognitive and Motor Performance Deficits during Sleep Deprivation," *Nutritional Neuroscience* 6, no. 4 (2003): 237–46; and David F. Neri et al., "The Effects of Tyrosine on Cognitive Performance during Extended Wakefulness," *Aviation, Space, and Environmental Medicine* 66, no. 4 (1995): 313–19.

133. "IUPHAR/BPS Guide to PHARMACOLOGY," International Union of Basic and Clinical Pharmacology, March 15, 2017, http://www.guidetoimmunopharmacology.org/immuno/index.jsp; and Yingxue Li et al., "Opioid Glycopeptide Analgesics Derived from Endogenous Enkephalins and Endorphins," *Future Medicinal Chemistry* 4, no. 2 (2012): 205–26.

134. R. R. W. J. van der Hulst et al., "Glutamine and the Preservation of Gut Integrity," *Lancet* 341, no. 8857 (1993): 1363–65; Fatma G. Huffman and Melanie E. Walgren, "L-Glutamine Supplementation Improves Nelfinavir-Associated Diarrhea in HIV-Infected Individuals," *HIV Clinical Trials* 4, no. 5 (2003): 324–29.

135. Jan Albrecht et al., "Roles of Glutamine in Neurotransmission," *Neuron Glia Biology* 6, no. 4 (2010): 263–76.

136. Itzhak Nissim et al., "Acid-Base Regulation of Hepatic Glutamine Metabolism and Ureagenesis: Study with 15N," *Journal of the American Society of Nephrology* 3, no. 7 (1993): 1416–27.

137. Zayd Merza, "Chronic Use of Opioids and the Endocrine System," *Hormone and Metabolic Research* 42, no. 9 (2010): 621–26; and J. A. Elliott, S. E. Opper, S. Agarwal, and E. E. Fibuch, "Non-analgesic Effects of Opioids: Opioids and the Endocrine System," *Current Pharmacology Discussion* 18, no. 37 (2012): 6070–78.

138. Alessandro Colasanti et al., "Opioids and Anxiety," *Journal of Psychopharmacology* 25, no. 11 (2011): 1415–33.

139. Robert M. Swift and Robert L. Stout, "The Relationship between Craving, Anxiety, and Other Symptoms in Opioid Withdrawal," *Journal of Substance Abuse* 4, no. 1 (1992): 19–26.

140. Rikita Merai et al., "CDC Grand Rounds: A Public Health Approach to Detect and Control Hypertension," *Morbidity and Mortality Weekly Report* 65, no. 45 (2016): 1261–64.

141. Dariush Mozzafarian et al., "Heart Disease and Stroke Statistics — 2015 Update: A Report from the American Heart Association," *Circulation* 131, no. 4 (January 27, 2015): e29–e322.

142. Howard S. Smith, "Opioid Metabolism," *Mayo Clinic Proceedings* 84, no. 7 (2009): 613–24.

143. Maria C. Mancebo et al., "Substance Use Disorders in an Obsessive Compulsive Disorder Clinical Sample," *Journal of Anxiety Disorders* 23, no. 4 (2009): 429–35; and Irit Friedman, Reuven Dar, and Etay Shilony, "Compulsivity and Obsessionality in Opioid Addiction," *Journal of Nervous and Mental Disease* 188, no. 3 (March 2000): 155–62.

144. Jane Liebschutz et al., "The Relationship between Sexual and Physical Abuse and Substance Abuse Consequences," *Journal of Substance Abuse Treatment* 22, no. 3 (2002): 121–28.

145. Courtney Lee et al., "The Effectiveness of Acupuncture Research across Components of the Trauma Spectrum Response (TSR): A Systematic Review of Reviews," *Systematic Reviews* 1, no. 46 (2012); Wayne B. Jonas et al., "A Randomized Exploratory Study to Evaluate Two Acupuncture Methods for the Treatment of Headaches Associated with Traumatic Brain Injury," *Medical Acupuncture* 28, no. 3 (2016): 113–30; and Charles C. Engel et al., "Randomized Effectiveness Trial of a Brief Course of Acupuncture for Posttraumatic Stress Disorder," *Medical Care* 52 (2014): S57–S64.

146. Mark A. Micek et al., "Complementary and Alternative Medicine Use among Veterans Affairs Outpatients," *Journal of Alternative and Complementary Medicine* 13, no. 2 (2007): 190–93.

147. F. Patricia McEachrane-Gross, Jane Liebschutz, and Dan Berlowitz, "Use of Selected Complementary and Alternative Medicine (CAM) Treatments in Veterans with Cancer or Chronic Pain: A Cross-Sectional Survey," *BMC Complementary and Alternative Medicine* 6, no. 34 (2006).

148. Barbara Goldberg, "Opioid Abuse Crisis Takes Heavy Toll on U.S. Veterans," Reuters, November 10, 2017, https://www.reuters.com/article/us-usa-veterans-opioids/opioid-abuse-crisis-takes-heavy-toll-on-u-s-veterans-idUSKBN1DA1B2; and Sarah Childress, "Veterans Face Greater Risks Amid Opioid Crisis," PBS Frontline, March 28, 2016, https://www.pbs.org/wgbh/frontline/article/veterans-face-greater-risks-amid-opioid-crisis/.

149. Thomas F. Northrup et al., "Opioid Withdrawal, Craving, and Use During and After Outpatient Buprenorphine Stabilization and Taper: A Discrete Survival and Growth Mixture Model," *Addictive Behaviors* 41 (February 2105): 20–28.

150. Sompon Wanwimolruk and Virapong Prachayasittikul, "Cytochrome P450 Enzyme Mediated Herbal Drug Interactions (Part 1)," *Experimental and Clinical Sciences Journal* 13 (2014): 347–91.

151. Lin Kang et al., "Tai-Kang-Ning, a Chinese Herbal Medicine Formula, Alleviates Acute Heroin Withdrawal," *American Journal of Drug and Alcohol Abuse* 34, no. 3 (2008): 269–76.

152. M. J. Christie, "Cellular Neuroadaptations to Chronic Opioids: Tolerance, Withdrawal and Addiction," *British Journal of Pharmacology* 154 (2008): 384–96; and Ashish K. Rehni, Amteshwar S. Jaggi, and Nirmal Singh, "Opioid Withdrawal Syndrome: Emerging Concepts and Novel Therapeutic Targets," *CNS & Neurological Disorders: Drug Targets* 12, no. 1 (2013): 112–25.

153. Christopher M. Jones, "Heroin Use and Heroin Use Risk Behaviors among Nonmedical Users of Prescription Opioid Pain Relievers: United States, 2002–2004 and 2008–2010," *Drug and Alcohol Dependence* 132, nos. 1–2 (2013): 95–100.

154. Elizabeth Llorente, "New Jersey's New Opioid Law Raises Concerns among Doctors," Fox News Health, May 9, 2017, http://www.foxnews.com/health/2017/05/09/new-jerseys-new-opioid-law-raises-concerns-among-doctors.html; and Eric Russell, "Legislators Urged to Clarify Opioid Law That Restricts Long-Term Use of Painkillers," *Portland Press Herald*, April 20, 2017, http://www.pressherald.com/2017/04/20/chronic-pain-patients-say-new-law-regulating-opioid-prescriptions-is-harming-them/.

155. Richard L. Nahin et al., "Evidence-Based Evaluation of Complementary Health Approaches for Pain Management in the United States," *Mayo Clinic Proceedings* 91, no. 9 (2016): 1292–306; María Villarreal Santiago et al., "Does Acupuncture Alter Pain-Related Functional Connectivity of the Central Nervous System? A Systematic Review," *Journal of Acupuncture and Meridian Studies* 9, no. 4 (2016): 167–77; and Alena Ondrejkovicova et al., "Why Acupuncture in Pain Treatment?," *Neuroendocrinology Letters* 37, no. 3 (2016): 163–68.

156. Li-Xin An et al., "Electro-Acupuncture Decreases Postoperative Pain and Improves Recovery in Patients Undergoing Supratentorial Craniotomy," *American Journal of Chinese Medicine* 42, no. 5 (2014): 1099–109; Chun-Chieh Chen et al., "Acupuncture for Pain Relief after Total Knee Arthroplasty: A Randomized Controlled Trial," *Regional Anesthesia and Pain Medicine* 40, no. 1 (2015): 31–36; Hye Kyung Cho et al., "Can Perioperative Acupuncture Reduce the Pain and Vomiting Experienced after Tonsillectomy? A Meta-Analysis," *Laryngoscope* 126, no. 3 (2016): 608–15; Young-Hun Cho et al., "Acupuncture for Acute Postoperative Pain after Back Surgery: A Systematic Review and Meta-Analysis of Randomized Controlled Trials," *Pain Practice* 15, no. 3 (2015): 279–91; and Daniel J. Crespin et al., "Acupuncture Provides Short-Term Pain Relief for Patients in a Total Joint Replacement Program," *Pain Medicine* 16, no. 6 (2015): 1195–203.

157. Leslie J. Crofford, "Chronic Pain: Where the Body Meets the Brain," *Transactions of the American Clinical and Climatological Association* 126 (2015): 167–83.

158. Chris Bleakley, Suzanne McDonough, and Domhnall MacAuley, "The Use of Ice in the Treatment of Acute Soft-Tissue Injury," *American Journal of Sports Medicine* 32, no. 1 (2004): 251–61.

159. D. Dent-Breen, "Rethinking RICE: The Old Standard Method May Not Actually Be the Best Treatment for Acute Injuries," EmaxHealth, July 12, 2017, https://www .emaxhealth.com/13737/rethinking-rice-old -standard-method-may-not-actually-be-best -treatment-acute-injuries.

160. P. Rapeli et al., "Cognitive Function during Early Abstinence from Opioid Dependence: A Comparison to Age, Gender, and Verbal Intelligence Matched Controls," *BMC Psychiatry* 6 (2006): 9.

161. "Many Fentanyl and Heroin Overdose Survivors Suffering Permanent Brain Damage," The Dunes East Hampton, March 3, 2017, https://theduneseasthampton .com/blog/many-fentanyl-and-heroin -overdose-survivors-suffering-permanent -brain-damage/.

162. Z. Merza, "Chronic Use of Opioids and the Endocrine System"; J. A. Elliott, S. E. Opper, S. Agarwal, and E. E. Fibuch, "Non-analgesic Effects of Opioids: Opioids and the Endocrine System" *Current Pharmacology Discussion* 18, no. 37 (2012): 6070–78; and Todd T. Brown, Amy B. Wisniewski, and Adrian S. Dobs, "Gonadal and Adrenal Abnormalities in Drug Users: Cause or Consequence of Drug Use Behavior and Poor Health Outcomes," *American Journal of Infectious Diseases* 2, no. 3 (2006): 130–35.

163. Andrew Ellis, *Fundamentals of Chinese Acupuncture*, rev. ed. (Brookline, MA: Paradigm, 1991).

164. Wojciech Leppert, "The Impact of Opioid Analgesics on the Gastrointestinal Tract Function and the Current Management Possibilities," *Contemporary Oncology* 16, no. 2 (2012): 125–31; and Peter Holzer, "Treatment of Opioid-Induced Gut Dysfunction," *Expert Opinion on Investigative Drugs* 16, no. 2 (2007): 181–94.

165. Ramsin Benyamin et al., "Opioid Complications and Side Effects," *Pain Physician* 11, no. 2S (2008): S105–S120.

166. Samira Alinejad et al., "A Systematic Review of the Cardiotoxicity of Methadone," *EXCLI Journal* 14 (May 5, 2015): 577–600; and Erich F. Wedam and Mark C. Haigney, "The Impact of Opioids on Cardiac Electrophysiology," *Current Cardiology Review* 12, no. 1 (2016): 27–36.

167. Mirsada Serdarevic et al., "The Association between Insomnia and Prescription Opioid Use: Results from a Community Sample in Northeast Florida," *Sleep Health* 3, no. 5 (2017): 368–72; and J. A. Robertson et al., "Sleep Disturbance in Patients Taking Opioid Medication for Chronic Back Pain," *Anaesthesia* 71, no. 11 (2016): 1296–307.

168. Hooman Khademi et al., "Opioid Therapy and Its Side Effects: A Review," *Archives of Iranian Medicine* 19, no. 12 (2016): 873.

169. Rajita Sinha, "Chronic Stress, Drug Use, and Vulnerability to Addiction," *Annals of the New York Academy of Sciences* 1141 (October 2008): 105.

Suggested Reading

Traditional Chinese Medicine

Beinfield, Harriet, and Efrem Korngold. *Between Heaven and Earth: A Guide to Chinese Medicine.* Random House, 1992.

Bensky, D. *Chinese Herbal Medicine: Formulas & Strategies.* Eastland Press, 1990.

Browne, Catherine. Class notes, Dragon Rises College, TCM graduate program and Five Branches University doctorate program, 1997–2017.

Chang, Chung-Ching. *Shang Han Lun: Wellspring of Chinese Medicine*, eds. Hong-yen Hsu and William G. Peacher. Oriental Healing Arts Institute, 1995.

Chen, John K., and Tina T. Chen. *Chinese Medical Herbology and Pharmacology.* Art of Medicine Press, 2003.

Connelly, Dianne M. *Traditional Acupuncture: The Law of the Five Elements*, 2nd ed. Traditional Acupuncture Institute, 1994.

De Morant, George Soulé. *Chinese Acupuncture.* Paradigm Publications, 1994.

Deng, Liang Yue. *Chinese Acupuncture and Moxibustion*, 6th ed. China Books & Periodicals, 1998.

Ellis, Andrew. *Fundamentals of Chinese Acupuncture.* Paradigm Publications, 1991.

Gaeddert, Andrew. *Chinese Herbs in the Western Clinic: A Guide to Prepared Herbal Formulas Indexed by Western Disorders & Supported by Case Studies.* Get Well Foundation, 1994.

Hammer, Leon. *Dragon Rises, Red Bird Flies: Psychology, Energy & Chinese Medicine.* Station Hill Press, 1991.

Hongtu, Wang. *Diseases, Symptoms, and Clinical Applications of Yellow Emperor's Canon of Internal Medicine*, ed. Richard R. Pearce. New World Press, 1999.

Hsu, Hong-Yen. *Oriental Materia Medica: A Concise Guide.* Oriental Healing Arts Institute, 1996.

Huang, Huang. *Ten Key Formula Families in Chinese Medicine.* Eastland Press, 2009.

Huihe, Yin. *Fundamentals of Traditional Chinese Medicine*, trans. Shuai Xue Zhong. Foreign Language Press, 1992.

Keys, John D. *Chinese Herbs: Their Botany, Chemistry, and Pharmacodynamics.* Tuttle Publishing, 1991.

Maciocia, Giovanni. *Obstetrics and Gynecology in Chinese Medicine.* Churchill Livingstone, 1998.

————. *The Practice of Chinese Medicine: The Treatment of Diseases with Acupuncture and Chinese Herbs,* 2nd ed. Churchill Livingstone, 2008.

Reid, Daniel P. *Chinese Herbal Medicine.* Shambhala, 1987.

Serizawa, Katsusuke. *Tsubo: Vital Points for Oriental Therapy.* Japan Publications, 1998.

Tierra, Lesley. *Herbs of Life: Health & Healing Using Western & Chinese Techniques.* Crossing Press, 1992.

Ohashi, Wataru. *Reading the Body: Ohashi's Book of Oriental Diagnosis.* Arkana, 1991.

Oleson, Terry. *Auriculotherapy Manual: Chinese and Western Systems of Ear Acupuncture,* 2nd ed. Health Care Alternatives, 1996.

Scott, John; Lorena Monda; and John Heuertz. *Clinical Guide to Commonly Used Chinese Herbal Formulas,* 5th ed. Herbal Medicine Press, 2006.

Xinghua, Bai. *Chinese Auricular Therapy.* Scientific & Technical Documents Publishing, 1994.

The Yellow Emperor's Classic of Medicine: A New Translation of the Neijing Suwen with Commentary, trans. Maoshing Ni. Shambhala Publications, 1995.

Western Herbals

Beale Galen, and Mary Rose Boswell. *The Earth Shall Blossom: Shaker Herbs and Gardening.* Countryman Press, 1999.

Christopher, John R. *School of Natural Healing.* Christopher Publications, 1996.

Crawford, Amanda McQuade. *Herbal Menopause Book: Herbs, Nutrition, & Other Natural Therapies.* Crossing Press, 1996.

Culpeper, Nicholas. *Culpeper's Color Herbal.* 1750; repr. Sterling, 1992.

Duke, James A. *The Green Pharmacy: New Discoveries in Herbal Remedies for Common Diseases and Conditions from the World's Foremost Authority on Healing Herbs.* Rodale, 1997.

Freeman, Sally. *EveryWoman's Guide to Natural Home Remedies.* Doubleday Direct, 1996.

Grieve, Mrs. [Margaret]. *A Modern Herbal: The Medicinal, Culinary, Cosmetic and Economic Properties, Cultivation and Folk-Lore of Herbs, Grasses, Fungi, Shrubs & Trees With All Their Modern Scientific Uses,* ed. Mrs. C. F. Leyel. 2 vols. 1931; repr. Dover Publications, 1971.

Heinerman, John. *Heinerman's Encyclopedia of Healing Herbs & Spices.* Prentice Hall, 1995.

Hoffmann, David. *An Elders' Herbal: Natural Techniques for Promoting Health & Vitality.* Healing Arts Press, 1993.

———. *The Herbal Handbook: A User's Guide to Medical Herbalism*. Healing Arts Press, 1998.

———. *The New Holistic Herbal (Health Workbooks)*. Element Books, 1990.

Holmes, Peter. *The Energetics of Western Herbs: Treatment Strategies Integrating Western & Oriental Herbal Medicine*, 3rd rev. ed. 2 vols. Snow Lotus Press, 1999.

Junius, Manfred M. *The Practical Handbook of Plant Alchemy: An Herbalist's Guide to Preparing Medicinal Essences, Tinctures, and Elixirs*. Healing Arts Press, 1985.

Kenner, Dan, and Yves Requena. *Botanical Medicine: A European Professional Perspective*. Paradigm, 1996.

Mabey, Richard. *The New Age Herbalist: How to Use Herbs for Healing Nutrition Body Care and Relaxation*. Simon & Schuster, 1988.

McIntyre, Anne. (1995) *The Complete Woman's Herbal: A manual of Healing Herbs and Nutrition for Personal Well-Being and Family Care*. Holt, 1995.

Meyer, Joseph E. *The Old Herb Doctor*, 2nd ed., rev. Meyerbooks, 1984.

Mills, Simon Y. *Out of the Earth: The Essential Book of Herbal Medicine*. Penguin, 1991.

Mindell, Earl. *Earl Mindell's Herb Bible*. Simon & Schuster, 1992.

Mowrey, Daniel B. *Herbal Tonic Therapies*. Wings Books, 1996.

Murray, Michael T. *The Healing Power of Herbs: The Enlightened Person's Guide to the Wonders of Medicinal Plants*. 2nd ed. Prima Lifestyles, 1992.

Nostradamus. *The Elixirs of Nostradamus: Nostradamus' Original Recipes for Elixirs, Scented Water, Beauty Potions and Sweetmeats*, ed. Knut Boeser. Moyer Bell, 1996.

Ody, Penelope. *The Complete Guide to Medicinal Herbs*. Dorling Kindersley, 1993.

Soule, Deb. *The Roots of Healing: A Woman's Book of Herbs*. Citadel Press, 1995.

Squier, Thomas Broken Bear, with Lauren David Peden. *Herbal Folk Medicine: An A to Z Guide*. Henry Holt, 1997.

Theiss, Barbara, and Peter Theiss. *The Family Herbal: A Guide to Natural Health Care for Yourself and Your Children from Europe's Leading Herbalists*. Healing Arts Press, 1989.

Tobyn, Graeme. *Culpeper's Medicine: A Practice of Western Holistic Medicine*. Element Books, 1997.

Todd, Jude C. *Jude's Herbal Home Remedies: Natural Health, Beauty & Home-Care Secrets*, 2nd ed. Llewellyn, 2002.

Vogel, Alfred. *The Nature Doctor: A Manual of Traditional and Complementary Medicine*. Keats, 1991.

Wood, Matthew. *Seven Herbs: Plants as Teachers*. North Atlantic Books, 1987.

Resources

Acupuncturists

To find a licensed acupuncturist in your area, go to Acufinder.com, an acupunturist referral service.

Bulk Herbs and Natural Products

Frontier Co-op
www.frontiercoop.com

Gaia Herbs
www.gaiaherbs.com

Herb Pharm
www.herb-pharm.com

Mountain Rose Herbs
www.mountainroseherbs.com

Nuherbs Co.
nuherbs.com

Spring Wind Herbs
https://springwind.com

Starwest Botanicals
www.starwest-botanicals.com

Wise Woman Herbals
https://wisewomanherbals.com

Chinese Herb Formulas

Ageless Herbs
https://agelessherbs.com

Dragon Herbs
www.dragonherbs.com

Herbalist & Alchemist
www.herbalist-alchemist.com

Pacific Herbs
www.pacherbs.com

Planetary Herbals
www.planetaryherbals.com

Swan Creek Farm
swancreekfarm.com

Flower Essences

FES Flowers
https://fesflowers.com

Swan Creek Farm
swancreekfarm.com

Index

Page numbers in *italic* indicate illustrations; numbers in **bold** indicate charts.

brain, *continued*

  perception of pain and, 182

  reward pathway of, 17

burdock (*Arctium lappa*), 81

C

California poppy (*Eschscholzia californica*), 81

Calm Mind formula, 176, **176**

cannabis (*Cannabis sativa*), 82

capsules, 76

carrier oils, 99

case studies

  Chinese vs. Western medicine, 21–22

  Fire element imbalance, 157–59

  Metal element imbalance, 168–170

  Water element imbalance, 146–48

  Wood element imbalance, 151–53

cedar (*Cedrus deodara*), 103

channels, acupoints and, 51

cherry plum, 116

chestnut bud, 116

Chicken Soup, Restorative, 132

Chinese herbs, 68

Chinese medicine, 12, 19–21. *See also* five elements; Traditional Chinese Medicine (TCM)

  "bone knitting," 184

  energies and, 23–26

  internal wind, 37

  memory/cognitive deficits, 195–96

  natural versus pharmaceutical therapies, 181

  opioid addiction and, 20–21

  Six Pathogenic Factors, 36

  Taoist beliefs and, 22–23

  Western medicine versus, 21–22

cinnamon leaf (*Cinnamomum cassia*), 103–4

clary sage (*Salvia sclarea*), 104

clove (*Eugenia caryophyllata*), 105

codonopsis (*Codonopsis pilosula*), 83

cognition, L-tyrosine and, 137

cognitive deficits. *See* memory

Conception Vessel (CV), 61

  CV acupoints, 61, *67, 118, 119*

conditioned association, 17

constipation, 203–4

  Opioid-Induced Constipation Relief, 204, **204**

contraindications

  blood-moving herbs and, 183

  prescription medication and, 175

coriander (*Coriandrum sativum*), 105

cravings

  GABA and, 136

  L-tyrosine and, 137

  self-treatment for, 178

cun, body measurement and, 51

cupping, 48

Curing Pills, 179

CV. *See* Conception Vessel

cypress (*Cupressus sempervirens*), 106

D

dampness. *See also* internal dampness

  chronic pain/stiffness due to, 191–92

  damp bi, 191

  Damp Bi Spray, 192–93

dandelion (*Taraxacum officinale*), 83–84

dang shen. *See* codonopsis

decoctions, 76–77

depression, 11, 115

detoxification

  herbs, **69**, 72

  L-glutamine and, 138

  rapid or gradual cessation, 46

  self-treatment for, 178

  TCM and, 21

diet. *See* nutrition

digestion

  L-glutamine and, 138

  L-tryptophan/5-HTP and, 136

digestive problems, 202–3

  constipation, 203–4

  Liver qi stagnation, severe, 203

  Spleen qi deficiency, digestion and, 203

G

Gallbladder (GB)
    GB acupoints, 54–55, *63*
    Wood element meridians, *63*
gamma-aminobutyric acid (GABA), 136
genetic factors, disease and, 37–38
geranium (*Pelargonium graveolens*), 108
ginger (*Zingiber officinale*), 109
glycerites, 78
gobo. *See* burdock
goji (*Lycium chinense*), 86
gou qi zi. *See* goji
grief, 165

H

hawthorn (*Crataegus* spp.), 86
health. *See also* wellness
    complications, recovery and, 18
    restoration of, following withdrawal,
        47
health problems, long-term, 194–211
    constipation, 203–4
    digestive problems, 202–3
    fatigue, 199–202
    heart damage, 205
    high blood pressure, 205
    immune stress, 206–8
    memory/cognitive deficits, 195–98
    skin issues, 209–10
    sleep issues, 205–6
    stress, 208–9
    sweating, excessive, 210–11
Heart (HT). *See also* Fire/Heart imbalances; Pericardium
    blood deficiency, food therapy for, 129
    damage to, 205
    health of, herbs for, **70**, 72
    HT 5 acupoints, 55–56, *64*, 122
    memory/cognitive deficits, 196
    meridians, Fire element, *64*
    Opioid Heart Tonic, 156, **156**
    qi deficiency fatigue, 201
    sleep issues and, 205–6

Heat-Clearing Trauma Spray, 188–89
herb(s), 68–69. *See also* medicinal herbs
    adaptogens, **69**, 71–72
    categories of actions, **69–70**
    Chinese, 68
    contraindications and, 183
    detoxification, **69**, 72
    heart health, **70**, 72
    immune support, **69**, 72
    liver health, 73
    lung health, **70**, 73
    medicinal, 79–97, 133
    nervines, **69**, 71
    opioid dependency and, 69–74
    pain relief, **70**, 72
    psychoactive, **70**, 73
    realistic expectations and, 74
    tonic, **69**, 71
Herbal Ice, 186–87
herbal medicine, 41
herbal remedies, 74–78
    capsules, 76
    contraindications and, 75
    decoctions, 76–77
    glycerites, 78
    infusions, 76–77
    making, at home, 78
    tablets, 76
    TCM formulas, 75
    tinctures, 77
herbal therapy, opioid replacement drugs
   and, 174
Herb Mix, Medicinal, 133
heroin, 14, 15, 16
    addicts, recovering, 39
    prescription painkillers and, 180
he shou wu. *See* fo-ti
high blood pressure, 205
ho wood (*Cinnamomum camphora*), 110
HT. *See* Heart
huang qi. *See* astragalus
hydrocodone, 14

Water element, *continued*
    essential oils and, **100**
    Kidneys, 31, *31*, 196
    meridians, acupoints and, *62*
    panic/anxiety and, 39–40
Water/Kidney imbalances
    case study, 146–48
    imbalance, 141–48
    Kidney yang deficiency, 144–45
    Kidney yin deficiency, 142
    Opioid Yang Tonic, 145, **145**
    Opioid Yin Tonic, 143, **143**
wei qi (defensive energy), 207
    Restore Wei Qi formula, 208, **208**
wellness. *See also* health
    Chinese medicine and, 19, 36, 38, 39
    diet and, 38
    emotional, 39
    mind, body and, 47, 115
    withdrawal and, 171
Western medicine
    Chinese medicine versus, 21–22
    herbal, 68
    natural versus pharmaceutical
        therapies, 181
    raw foods and, 124
    RICE (rest, ice, compression,
        elevation), 187
white peony (*Paeonia laciflora*), 95
wild lettuce (*Lactuca virosa*), 95–96
wild rose, 117
willow (*Salix alba*), 96
withdrawal, 171–79
    acupuncture for, 45–47
    Calm Mind formula, 176, **176**
    Ease Detox formula, 177, **177**
    formulas, three primary, 174–77
    health restoration following, 47
    muscle cramps/spasms, 179
    natural therapies and, 11

opioid withdrawal syndrome, 171
    planning for success and, 172–73
    Quell Quease formula, 175, **175**
    relapse and, 9, 11, 21, 46, 174
    self-treatment options, 178–79
    skin itchiness and, 209
    weaning off/quitting cold turkey, 173
Wood element
    case study, imbalance, 151–53
    essential oils and, **100**
    Liver, 32, *32*, 196
    meridians, acupoints and, 63
    violence/suicide and, 40
Wood/Liver imbalances, 148–153
    Liver qi stagnation, 149
    Opioid Liver Balancer, 150, **150**
worthlessness/feeling trapped, Earth
    element and, 40–41
wu jia pi. *See* eleuthero
wu wei zi. *See* schisandra

Y

yang. *See* yin and yang
yang deficiency, 24
    Kidney, 31, 144
    Opioid Yang Tonic, 145, **145**
yarrow (*Achillea millefolium*), 96
yellow dock (*Rumex crispus*), 97
yi (intellect), 40
yin and yang, 23–24, 24. *See also* yang
    deficiency
    yin organs/yang organs, 29
yin deficiency, 23–24
    dry skin and, 210
    Kidney, 142–43, **143**, 211

Z

zinc, 135